This *Medical Language Instant Translator* provides quick access to useful, medically related information for both laypersons and students entering health-related professions. Today we are increasingly exposed to medical terminology, whether it be at the doctor's office, on the Internet, or in the media. Analyzing and understanding these terms allow us to participate in important issues affecting our society, as well as to make better decisions about our own health.

Using this handy pocket-sized book, you will be able to:

- Decipher complicated medical terms by recognizing and finding the meanings of individual word parts
- Distinguish between commonly misunderstood medical terms
- Recognize specialized terms used in medical records
- Access information on medical abbreviations, symbols, acronyms, and professional designations
- Understand the definitions of commonly used diagnostic tests and procedures
- Identify the top 100 prescription drugs and their uses
- Understand the significance of familiar complementary and alternative medicine terms
- Interpret the significance of common blood tests
- Visualize the location of many organs and body structures with full-color illustrations

Although this *Instant Translator* dovetails with information in both my books, *The Language of Medicine* and *Medical Terminology: A Short Course*, all students of medical language can benefit from it. Please let me know how the *Instant Translator* works for you. Have fun using it!

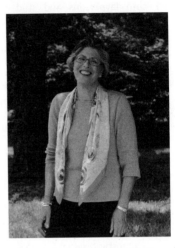

Davi-Ellen Chabner
MedDavi@aol.com

DAVI-ELLEN CHABNER, BA, MAT

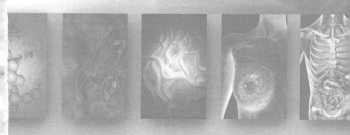

Medical Language
Instant
Translator

FOURTH EDITION

SAUNDERS
ELSEVIER

3251 Riverport Lane
Maryland Heights, Missouri 63043

**MEDICAL LANGUAGE INSTANT
TRANSLATOR, FOURTH EDITION**   ISBN: 978-1-4377-0564-5

Notices

ISBN: 978-1-4377-0564-5

Publisher: Jeanne Olson
Senior Developmental Editor: Becky Swisher
Publishing Services Manager: Patricia Tannian
Senior Project Manager: John Casey
Senior Designer: Ellen Zanolle

Printed in United States of America

Last digit is the print number: 9   8   7   6   5   4   3

Contents

v

PART 3   Body Systems Illustrations

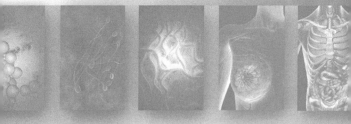

PART 1

The Language
of Medicine

How to Analyze Medical Terms*

Studying medical terminology is very similar to learning a new language. At first, the words sound strange and complicated, although they may stand for commonly known disorders and terms. For example, **cephalgia** means "headache," and an **ophthalmologist** is an "eye doctor."

Your first job in learning the language of medicine is to understand how to divide words into their component parts. Logically, most terms, whether complex or simple, can be broken down into basic parts and then understood. For example, consider the following term:

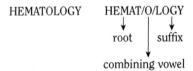

The **root** is the *foundation of the word*. All medical terms have one or more roots. For example, the root **hemat** means **blood**.

The **suffix** is the *word ending*. All medical terms have a suffix. The suffix **-logy** means **process of study**.

The **combining vowel**—usually **o**, as in this term—*links the root to the suffix or the root to another root*. A combining vowel has no meaning of its own; it joins one word part to another.

It is useful to read the meaning of medical terms *starting from the suffix and then going back to the beginning of the term*. Thus, the term **hematology** means **process of study of blood**.

---

*From Chabner DE: The Language of Medicine, 9th ed. Philadelphia, Saunders, 2011.

Here is another familiar medical term:

ELECTROCARDIOGRAM   ELECTR/O/CARDI/O/GRAM

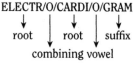

The root **electr** means electricity.
The root **cardi** means **heart**.
The suffix **-gram** means **record**.
The entire word (reading from the suffix back to the beginning of the term) means **record of the electricity in the heart**.

Notice that there are two combining vowels—both **o**—in this term. The first o links the two roots **electr** and **cardi**; the second o links the root **cardi** and the suffix **-gram**.

Try another term:

GASTRITIS   GASTR/ITIS
              ↓   ↓
            root suffix

The root **gastr** means **stomach**.
The suffix **-itis** means **inflammation**.
The entire word, reading from the end of the term (suffix) to the beginning, means **inflammation of the stomach**.

Notice that the combining vowel, o, is missing in this term. This is because the suffix, **-itis**, begins with a vowel. The combining vowel is dropped before a suffix that begins with a vowel. It is retained, however, between two roots, even if the second root begins with a vowel. Consider the following term:

GASTROENTEROLOGY   GASTR/O/ENTER/O/LOGY

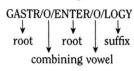

The root **gastr** means **stomach**.
The root **enter** means **intestines**.
The suffix **-logy** means **process of study**.
The entire term means **process of study of the stomach and intestines**.

Notice that the combining vowel is used between **gastr** and **enter**, even though the second root, **enter**, begins with a vowel. When a term contains two or more roots related to parts of the body, anatomic position often determines which root goes before the other. For example, the stomach receives food first, before the small intestine—so the word is formed as **gastroenterology**, not "enterogastrology."

In summary, remember three general rules:
1. Read the meaning of medical terms from the suffix back to the beginning of the term and across.
2. Drop the combining vowel (usually o) before a suffix beginning with a vowel: **gastritis**, *not* "gastroitis."
3. Keep the combining vowel between two roots: **gastroenterology**, *not* "gastrenterology."

In addition to the root, suffix, and combining vowel, two other word parts are commonly found in medical terms. These are the **combining form** and the **prefix**. The combining form is simply the root plus the combining vowel. For example, you already are familiar with the following combining forms and their meanings:

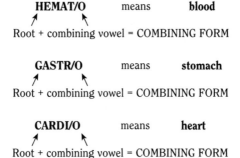

HEMAT/O   means   **blood**

Root + combining vowel = COMBINING FORM

GASTR/O   means   **stomach**

Root + combining vowel = COMBINING FORM

CARDI/O   means   **heart**

Root + combining vowel = COMBINING FORM

Combining forms are used with many different suffixes. Remembering the meaning of a combining form will help you understand different medical terms.

The **prefix** is a small part that is attached to the *beginning of a term*. Not all medical terms contain prefixes, but the prefix can have an important influence on the meaning. Consider the following examples:

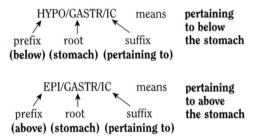

HYPO/GASTR/IC   means   **pertaining to below the stomach**

prefix   root   suffix
(below) (stomach) (pertaining to)

EPI/GASTR/IC   means   **pertaining to above the stomach**

prefix   root   suffix
(above) (stomach) (pertaining to)

In summary, the important elements of medical terms are the following:

1. **Root**: foundation of the term
2. **Suffix**: word ending
3. **Prefix**: word beginning
4. **Combining vowel**: vowel (usually o) that links the root to the suffix or the root to another root
5. **Combining form**: combination of the root and the combining vowel

Glossary of Word Parts Used in Medical Terminology*

MEDICAL WORD PARTS—ENGLISH

COMBINING FORM, SUFFIX, OR PREFIX	MEANING
a-, an-	no; not; without
ab-	away from
abdomin/o	abdomen
-ac	pertaining to
acanth/o	spiny; thorny
acetabul/o	acetabulum (hip socket)
acous/o	hearing
acr/o	extremities; top; extreme point
acromi/o	acromion (extension of shoulder bone)
actin/o	light
acu/o	sharp; severe; sudden
-acusis	hearing
ad-	toward
-ad	toward
aden/o	gland
adenoid/o	adenoids
adip/o	fat
adren/o	adrenal gland
adrenal/o	adrenal gland
aer/o	air
af-	toward
agglutin/o	clumping; sticking together

---

*From Chabner DE: The Language of Medicine, 9th ed. Philadelphia, Saunders, 2011.

MEDICAL WORD PARTS—ENGLISH
(Continued)

COMBINING FORM, SUFFIX, OR PREFIX	MEANING
-agon	assemble, gather
agora-	marketplace
-agra	excessive pain
-al	pertaining to
alb/o	white
albin/o	white
albumin/o	albumin (protein)
alges/o	sensitivity to pain
-algesia	sensitivity to pain
-algia	pain
all/o	other
alveol/o	alveolus; air sac; small sac
ambly/o	dim; dull
-amine	nitrogen compound
amni/o	amnion (sac surrounding the embryo)
amyl/o	starch
an/o	anus
-an	pertaining to
ana-	up; apart; backward; again, anew
andr/o	male
aneurysm/o	aneurysm (widened blood vessel)
angi/o	vessel (blood)
anis/o	unequal
ankyl/o	stiff
ante-	before; forward
anter/o	front
anthrac/o	coal
anthr/o	antrum of the stomach
anti-	against
anxi/o	uneasy; anxious
aort/o	aorta (largest artery)
-apheresis	removal

MEDICAL WORD PARTS—ENGLISH
(Continued)

COMBINING FORM, SUFFIX, OR PREFIX	MEANING
aphth/o	ulcer
apo-	off, away
aponeur/o	aponeurosis (type of tendon)
append/o	appendix
appendic/o	appendix
aque/o	water
-ar	pertaining to
-arche	beginning
arter/o	artery
arteri/o	artery
arteriol/o	arteriole (small artery)
arthr/o	joint
-arthria	articulate (speak distinctly)
articul/o	joint
-ary	pertaining to
asbest/o	asbestos
-ase	enzyme
-asthenia	lack of strength
atel/o	incomplete
ather/o	plaque (fatty substance)
-ation	process; condition
atri/o	atrium (upper heart chamber)
audi/o	hearing
audit/o	hearing
aur/o	ear
auricul/o	ear
aut/o	self, own
aut-, auto-	self, own
axill/o	armpit
azot/o	urea; nitrogen
bacill/o	bacilli (bacteria)
bacteri/o	bacteria
balan/o	glans penis
bar/o	pressure; weight

MEDICAL WORD PARTS—ENGLISH
(Continued)

COMBINING FORM, SUFFIX, OR PREFIX	MEANING
bartholin/o	Bartholin glands
bas/o	base; opposite of acid
bi-	two
bi/o	life
bil/i	bile; gall
bilirubin/o	bilirubin
-blast	embryonic; immature cell
-blastoma	immature tumor (cells)
blephar/o	eyelid
bol/o	cast; throw
brachi/o	arm
brachy-	short
brady-	slow
bronch/o	bronchial tube
bronchi/o	bronchial tube
bronchiol/o	bronchiole
bucc/o	cheek
bunion/o	bunion
burs/o	bursa (sac of fluid near joints)
byssin/o	cotton dust
cac/o	bad
calc/o	calcium
calcane/o	calcaneus (heel bone)
calci/o	calcium
cali/o	calyx
calic/o	calyx
capillar/o	capillary (tiniest blood vessel)
capn/o	carbon dioxide
-capnia	carbon dioxide
carcin/o	cancerous; cancer
cardi/o	heart
carp/o	wrist bones (carpals)
cata-	down
caud/o	tail; lower part of body
caus/o	burn; burning

MEDICAL WORD PARTS—ENGLISH
(Continued)

COMBINING FORM, SUFFIX, OR PREFIX	MEANING
cauter/o	heat; burn
cec/o	cecum (first part of the colon)
-cele	hernia
celi/o	belly; abdomen
-centesis	surgical puncture to remove fluid
cephal/o	head
cerebell/o	cerebellum (posterior part of the brain)
cerebr/o	cerebrum (largest part of the brain)
cerumin/o	cerumen
cervic/o	neck; cervix (neck of uterus)
-chalasia	relaxation
-chalasis	relaxation
cheil/o	lip
chem/o	drug; chemical
-chezia	defecation; elimination of wastes
chir/o	hand
chlor/o	green
chlorhydr/o	hydrochloric acid
chol/e	bile; gall
cholangi/o	bile vessel
cholecyst/o	gallbladder
choledoch/o	common bile duct
cholesterol/o	cholesterol
chondr/o	cartilage
chore/o	dance
chori/o	chorion (outermost membrane of the fetus)
chorion/o	chorion
choroid/o	choroid layer of eye
chrom/o	color
chron/o	time

MEDICAL WORD PARTS—ENGLISH
(Continued)

COMBINING FORM, SUFFIX, OR PREFIX	MEANING
chym/o	to pour
cib/o	meal
-cide	killing
-cidal	pertaining to killing
cine/o	movement
cirrh/o	orange-yellow
cis/o	to cut
-clasis	to break
-clast	to break
claustr/o	enclosed space
clavicul/o	clavicle (collar bone)
-clysis	irrigation; washing
coagul/o	coagulation (clotting)
-coccus (-cocci, *pl.*)	berry-shaped bacterium
coccyg/o	coccyx (tailbone)
cochle/o	cochlea (inner part of ear)
col/o	colon (large intestine)
coll/a	glue
colon/o	colon (large intestine)
colp/o	vagina
comat/o	deep sleep
comi/o	to care for
con-	together, with
coni/o	dust
conjunctiv/o	conjunctiva (lines the eyelids)
-constriction	narrowing
contra-	against; opposite
cor/o	pupil
core/o	pupil
corne/o	cornea
coron/o	heart
corpor/o	body
cortic/o	cortex, outer region

MEDICAL WORD PARTS—ENGLISH
(Continued)

COMBINING FORM, SUFFIX, OR PREFIX	MEANING
cost/o	rib
crani/o	skull
cras/o	mixture; temperament
crin/o	secrete
-crine	secrete; to separate
-crit	separate
cry/o	cold
crypt/o	hidden
culd/o	cul-de-sac
-cusis	hearing
cutane/o	skin
cyan/o	blue
cycl/o	ciliary body of eye; cycle; circle
-cyesis	pregnancy
cyst/o	urinary bladder; cyst; sac of fluid
cyt/o	cell
-cyte	cell
-cytosis	condition of cells; slight increase in numbers
dacry/o	tear
dacryoaden/o	tear gland
dacryocyst/o	tear sac; lacrimal sac
dactyl/o	fingers; toes
de-	lack of; down; less; removal of
dem/o	people
dent/i	tooth
derm/o	skin
-derma	skin
dermat/o	skin
desicc/o	drying
-desis	bind, tie together
dia-	complete; through

MEDICAL WORD PARTS—ENGLISH
(Continued)

COMBINING FORM, SUFFIX, OR PREFIX	MEANING
diaphor/o	sweat
-dilation	widening; stretching; expanding
dipl/o	double
dips/o	thirst
dist/o	far; distant
dors/o	back (of body)
dorsi-	back
-dote	to give
-drome	to run
duct/o	to lead, carry
duoden/o	duodenum
dur/o	dura mater
-dynia	pain
dys-	bad; painful; difficult; abnormal
-eal	pertaining to
ec-	out; outside
echo-	reflected sound
-ectasia	dilation; dilatation; widening
-ectasis	dilation; dilatation; widening
ecto-	out; outside
-ectomy	removal; excision; resection
-edema	swelling
-elasma	flat plate
electr/o	electricity
em-	in
-ema	condition
-emesis	vomiting
-emia	blood condition
-emic	pertaining to blood condition
emmetr/o	in due measure
en-	in; within
encephal/o	brain
end-	in; within
endo-	in; within

MEDICAL WORD PARTS—ENGLISH
(Continued)

COMBINING FORM, SUFFIX, OR PREFIX	MEANING
enter/o	intestines (usually small intestine)
eosin/o	red; rosy; dawn-colored
epi-	above; upon; on
epididym/o	epididymis
epiglott/o	epiglottis
episi/o	vulva (external female genitalia)
epitheli/o	skin; epithelium
equin/o	horse
-er	one who
erg/o	work
erythem/o	flushed; redness
erythr/o	red
-esis	action; condition; state of
eso-	inward
esophag/o	esophagus
esthes/o	nervous sensation (feeling)
esthesi/o	nervous sensation
-esthesia	nervous sensation
estr/o	female
ethm/o	sieve
eti/o	cause
eu-	good; normal
-eurysm	widening
ex-	out; away from
exanthemat/o	rash
exo-	out; away from
extra-	outside
faci/o	face
fasci/o	fascia (membrane supporting muscles)
femor/o	femur (thigh bone)
-ferent	to carry
fibr/o	fiber

MEDICAL WORD PARTS—ENGLISH
(Continued)

COMBINING FORM, SUFFIX, OR PREFIX	MEANING
fibros/o	fibrous connective tissue
fibul/o	fibula
-fication	process of making
-fida	split
flex/o	bend
fluor/o	luminous
follicul/o	follicle; small sac
-form	resembling; in the shape of
fung/i	fungus; mushroom (lower organism lacking chlorophyll)
furc/o	forking; branching
-fusion	to pour; to come together
galact/o	milk
ganglion/o	ganglion; collection of nerve cell bodies
gastr/o	stomach
-gen	substance that produces
-genesis	producing; forming
-genic	produced by or in
ger/o	old age
geront/o	old age
gest/o	pregnancy
gester/o	pregnancy
gingiv/o	gum
glauc/o	gray
gli/o	glial cells; neuroglial cells (supportive tissue of nervous system)
-globin	protein
-globulin	protein
glomerul/o	glomerulus
gloss/o	tongue
gluc/o	glucose; sugar
glyc/o	glucose; sugar
glycogen/o	glycogen; animal starch

MEDICAL WORD PARTS—ENGLISH
(Continued)

COMBINING FORM, SUFFIX, OR PREFIX	MEANING
glycos/o	glucose; sugar
gnos/o	knowledge
gon/o	seed
gonad/o	sex glands
goni/o	angle
-grade	to go
-gram	record
granul/o	granule(s)
-graph	instrument for recording
-graphy	process of recording
gravid/o	pregnancy
-gravida	pregnant woman
gynec/o	woman; female
hallucin/o	hallucination
hem/o	blood
hemat/o	blood
hemi-	half
hemoglobin/o	hemoglobin
hepat/o	liver
herni/o	hernia
-hexia	state of
hidr/o	sweat
hist/o	tissue
histi/o	tissue
home/o	sameness; unchanging; constant
hormon/o	hormone
humer/o	humerus (upper arm bone)
hydr/o	water
hyper-	above; excessive
hypn/o	sleep
hypo-	deficient; below; under; less than normal
hypophys/o	pituitary gland
hyster/o	uterus; womb

MEDICAL WORD PARTS—ENGLISH
(Continued)

COMBINING FORM, SUFFIX, OR PREFIX	MEANING
-ia	condition
-iac	pertaining to
-iasis	abnormal condition
iatr/o	physician; treatment
-ic	pertaining to
-ical	pertaining to
ichthy/o	dry; scaly
-icle	small
idi/o	unknown; individual; distinct
-ile	pertaining to
ile/o	ileum
ili/o	ilium
immun/o	immune; protection; safe
in-	in; into; not
-in, -ine	a substance
-ine	pertaining to
infra-	below; inferior to; beneath
inguin/o	groin
insulin/o	insulin (pancreatic hormone)
inter-	between
intra-	within; into
iod/o	iodine
ion/o	ion; to wander
-ion	process
-ior	pertaining to
ipsi-	same
ir-	in
ir/o	iris (colored portion of eye)
irid/o	iris (colored portion of eye)
is/o	same; equal
isch/o	hold back; back
ischi/o	ischium (part of hip bone)
-ism	process; condition
-ist	specialist
-itis	inflammation
-itus	condition
-ium	structure; tissue

MEDICAL WORD PARTS—ENGLISH
(Continued)

COMBINING FORM, SUFFIX, OR PREFIX	MEANING
jaund/o	yellow
jejun/o	jejunum
kal/i	potassium
kary/o	nucleus
kerat/o	cornea; hard, horny tissue
kern-	nucleus (collection of nerve cells in the brain)
ket/o	ketones; acetones
keton/o	ketones; acetones
kines/o	movement
kinesi/o	movement
-kinesia	movement
-kinesis	movement
klept/o	to steal
kyph/o	humpback
labi/o	lip
lacrim/o	tear; tear duct; lacrimal duct
lact/o	milk
lamin/o	lamina (part of vertebral arch)
lapar/o	abdominal wall; abdomen
-lapse	slide, fall, sag
laryng/o	larynx (voice box)
later/o	side
leiomy/o	smooth (visceral) muscle
-lemma	sheath, covering
-lepsy	seizure
lept/o	thin, slender
-leptic	pertaining to seizing, taking hold of
leth/o	death
leuk/o	white
lex/o	word; phrase
-lexia	word; phrase
ligament/o	ligament

MEDICAL WORD PARTS—ENGLISH
(Continued)

COMBINING FORM, SUFFIX, OR PREFIX	MEANING
lingu/o	tongue
lip/o	fat; lipid
-listhesis	slipping
lith/o	stone; calculus
-lithiasis	condition of stones
-lithotomy	incision (for removal) of a stone
lob/o	lobe
log/o	study
-logy	study (process of)
lord/o	curve; swayback
-lucent	to shine
lumb/o	lower back; loin
lute/o	yellow
lux/o	slide
lymph/o	lymph
lymphaden/o	lymph gland (node)
lymphangi/o	lymph vessel
-lysis	breakdown; separation; destruction; loosening
-lytic	reducing, destroying; separating; breakdown
macro-	large
mal-	bad
-malacia	softening
malleol/o	malleolus
mamm/o	breast
mandibul/o	mandible (lower jaw bone)
-mania	obsessive preoccupation
mast/o	breast
mastoid/o	mastoid process (behind the ear)
maxill/o	maxilla (upper jaw bone)
meat/o	meatus (opening)
medi/o	middle
mediastin/o	mediastinum

MEDICAL WORD PARTS—ENGLISH
(Continued)

COMBINING FORM, SUFFIX, OR PREFIX	MEANING
medull/o	medulla (inner section); middle; soft, marrow
mega-	large
-megaly	enlargement
melan/o	black
men/o	menses; menstruation
mening/o	meninges (membranes covering the spinal cord and brain)
meningi/o	meninges
ment/o	mind; chin
meso-	middle
meta-	change; beyond
metacarp/o	metacarpals (hand bones)
metatars/o	metatarsals (foot bones)
-meter	measure
metr/o	uterus (womb); measure
metri/o	uterus (womb)
mi/o	smaller; less
micro-	small
-mimetic	mimic; copy
-mission	send
mon/o	one; single
morph/o	shape; form
mort/o	death
-mortem	death
-motor	movement
muc/o	mucus
mucos/o	mucous membrane (mucosa)
multi-	many
mut/a	genetic change
mutagen/o	causing genetic change
my/o	muscle
myc/o	fungus
mydr/o	wide
myel/o	spinal cord; bone marrow

MEDICAL WORD PARTS—ENGLISH
(Continued)

COMBINING FORM, SUFFIX, OR PREFIX	MEANING
myocardi/o	myocardium (heart muscle)
myom/o	muscle tumor
myos/o	muscle
myring/o	tympanic membrane (eardrum)
myx/o	mucus
narc/o	numbness; stupor; sleep
nas/o	nose
nat/i	birth
natr/o	sodium
necr/o	death
nect/o	bind, tie, connect
neo-	new
nephr/o	kidney
neur/o	nerve
neutr/o	neither; neutral; neutrophil
nid/o	nest
noct/o	night
norm/o	rule; order
nos/o	disease
nucle/o	nucleus
nulli-	none
nyct/o	night
obstetr/o	pregnancy; childbirth
ocul/o	eye
odont/o	tooth
odyn/o	pain
-oid	resembling; derived from
-ole	little; small
olecran/o	olecranon (elbow)
olig/o	scanty
om/o	shoulder
-oma	tumor; mass; fluid collection
omphal/o	umbilicus (navel)
onc/o	tumor

MEDICAL WORD PARTS—ENGLISH
(Continued)

COMBINING FORM, SUFFIX, OR PREFIX	MEANING
-one	hormone
onych/o	nail (of fingers or toes)
o/o	egg
oophor/o	ovary
-opaque	obscure
ophthalm/o	eye
-opia	vision condition
-opsia	vision condition
-opsy	view of
opt/o	eye; vision
optic/o	eye; vision
-or	one who
or/o	mouth
orch/o	testis
orchi/o	testis
orchid/o	testis
-orexia	appetite
orth/o	straight
-ose	full of; pertaining to; sugar
-osis	condition, usually abnormal
-osmia	smell
ossicul/o	ossicle (small bone)
oste/o	bone
-ostosis	condition of bone
ot/o	ear
-otia	ear condition
-ous	pertaining to
ov/o	egg
ovari/o	ovary
ovul/o	egg
ox/o	oxygen
-oxia	oxygen
oxy-	rapid; sharp; acid
oxysm/o	sudden

MEDICAL WORD PARTS—ENGLISH
(Continued)

COMBINING FORM, SUFFIX, OR PREFIX	MEANING
pachy-	heavy; thick
palat/o	palate (roof of the mouth)
palpebr/o	eyelid
pan-	all
pancreat/o	pancreas
papill/o	nipple-like; optic disc (disk)
par-	other than; abnormal
para-	near; beside; abnormal; apart from; along the side of
-para	to bear, bring forth (live births)
-parous	to bear, bring forth
parathyroid/o	parathyroid glands
-paresis	weakness
-pareunia	sexual intercourse
-partum	birth; labor
patell/a	patella
patell/o	patella
path/o	disease
-pathy	disease; emotion
pector/o	chest
ped/o	child; foot
pelv/i	pelvis; hip region
pelv/o	pelvis; hip region
pend/o	hang
-penia	deficiency
pen/o	penis
-pepsia	digestion
per-	through
peri-	surrounding
perine/o	perineum
peritone/o	peritoneum
perone/o	fibula
-pexy	fixation; to put in place
phac/o	lens of eye
phag/o	eat; swallow
-phage	eat; swallow

MEDICAL WORD PARTS—ENGLISH
(Continued)

COMBINING FORM, SUFFIX, OR PREFIX	MEANING
-phagia	condition of eating; swallowing
phak/o	lens of eye
phalang/o	phalanges (of fingers and toes)
phall/o	penis
pharmac/o	drug
pharmaceut/o	drug
pharyng/o	throat (pharynx)
phas/o	speech
-phasia	speech
phe/o	dusky; dark
-pheresis	removal
phil/o	like; love; attraction to
-phil	attraction for
-philia	attraction for
phim/o	muzzle
phleb/o	vein
phob/o	fear
-phobia	fear
phon/o	voice; sound
-phonia	voice; sound
phor/o	to bear
-phoresis	carrying; transmission
-phoria	to bear, carry; feeling (mental state)
phot/o	light
phren/o	diaphragm; mind
-phthisis	wasting away
-phylaxis	protection
physi/o	nature; function
-physis	to grow
phyt/o	plant
-phyte	plant
pil/o	hair
pineal/o	pineal gland

MEDICAL WORD PARTS—ENGLISH
(Continued)

COMBINING FORM, SUFFIX, OR PREFIX	MEANING
pituitar/o	pituitary gland
-plakia	plaque
plant/o	sole of the foot
plas/o	development; formation; growth
-plasia	development; formation; growth
-plasm	formation; structure
-plastic	pertaining to formation
-plasty	surgical repair
ple/o	more; many; varied
-plegia	paralysis; palsy
-plegic	pertaining to paralysis, palsy
pleur/o	pleura
plex/o	plexus; network (of nerves)
-pnea	breathing
pneum/o	lung; air; gas
pneumon/o	lung; air; gas
pod/o	foot
-poiesis	formation
-poietin	substance that forms
poikil/o	varied; irregular
pol/o	extreme
polio-	gray matter (of brain or spinal cord)
poly-	many; much
polyp/o	polyp; small growth
pont/o	pons (a part of the brain)
-porosis	condition of pores (spaces)
post-	after; behind
poster/o	back (of body); behind
-prandial	pertaining to eating or mealtime
-praxia	action
pre-	before; in front of
presby/o	old age

MEDICAL WORD PARTS—ENGLISH
(Continued)

COMBINING FORM, SUFFIX, OR PREFIX	MEANING
primi-	first
pro-	before; forward
proct/o	anus and rectum
pros-	before; forward
prostat/o	prostate gland
prot/o	first
prote/o	protein
proxim/o	near
prurit/o	itching
pseudo-	false
psych/o	mind
-ptosis	falling; drooping; prolapse
-ptysis	spitting
pub/o	pubis (anterior part of hip bone)
pulmon/o	lung
pupill/o	pupil (dark center of the eye)
purul/o	pus
py/o	pus
pyel/o	renal pelvis
pylor/o	pylorus; pyloric sphincter
pyr/o	fever; fire
pyret/o	fever
pyrex/o	fever
quadri-	four
rachi/o	spinal column; vertebrae
radi/o	x-rays; radioactivity; radius (lateral lower arm bone)
radicul/o	nerve root
re-	back; again; backward
rect/o	rectum
ren/o	kidney
reticul/o	network
retin/o	retina
retro-	behind; back; backward

MEDICAL WORD PARTS—ENGLISH
(Continued)

COMBINING FORM, SUFFIX, OR PREFIX	MEANING
rhabdomy/o	striated (skeletal) muscle
rheumat/o	watery flow
rhin/o	nose
rhytid/o	wrinkle
roentgen/o	x-rays
-rrhage	bursting forth (of blood)
-rrhagia	bursting forth (of blood)
-rrhaphy	suture
-rrhea	flow; discharge
-rrhexis	rupture
rrhythm/o	rhythm
sacr/o	sacrum
salping/o	fallopian tube; auditory (eustachian) tube
-salpinx	fallopian tube; oviduct
sarc/o	flesh (connective tissue)
scapul/o	scapula; shoulder blade
-schisis	split
schiz/o	split
scint/i	spark
scirrh/o	hard
scler/o	sclera (white of eye); hard
-sclerosis	hardening
scoli/o	crooked; bent
-scope	instrument for visual examination
-scopy	visual examination
scot/o	darkness
seb/o	sebum
sebace/o	sebum
sect/o	to cut
semi-	half
semin/i	semen; seed
seps/o	infection
sial/o	saliva
sialaden/o	salivary gland

MEDICAL WORD PARTS—ENGLISH
(Continued)

COMBINING FORM, SUFFIX, OR PREFIX	MEANING
sider/o	iron
sigmoid/o	sigmoid colon
silic/o	glass
sinus/o	sinus
-sis	state of; condition
-sol	solution
somat/o	body
-some	body
somn/o	sleep
-somnia	sleep
son/o	sound
-spadia	to tear, cut
-spasm	sudden contraction of muscles
sperm/o	spermatozoa; sperm cells
spermat/o	spermatozoa; sperm cells
sphen/o	wedge; sphenoid bone
spher/o	globe-shaped; round
sphygm/o	pulse
-sphyxia	pulse
splanchn/o	viscera (internal organs)
spin/o	spine (backbone)
spir/o	to breathe
splen/o	spleen
spondyl/o	vertebra (backbone)
squam/o	scale
-stalsis	contraction
staped/o	stapes (middle ear bone)
staphyl/o	clusters; uvula
-stasis	stopping; controlling; placing
-static	pertaining to stopping; controlling
steat/o	fat, sebum
sten/o	narrowing
-stenosis	tightening; stricture
ster/o	solid structure; steroid
stere/o	solid; three-dimensional

MEDICAL WORD PARTS—ENGLISH
(Continued)

COMBINING FORM, SUFFIX, OR PREFIX	MEANING
stern/o	sternum (breastbone)
steth/o	chest
-sthenia	strength
-stitial	pertaining to standing; positioned
stomat/o	mouth
-stomia	condition of the mouth
-stomy	new opening (to form a mouth)
strept/o	twisted chains
styl/o	pole or stake
sub-	under; below
submaxill/o	mandible (lower jaw bone)
-suppression	stopping
supra-	above, upper
sym-	together; with
syn-	together; with
syncop/o	to cut off, cut short; faint
syndesm/o	ligament
synov/o	synovia; synovial membrane; sheath around a tendon
syring/o	tube
tachy-	fast
tars/o	tarsus; hindfoot or ankle (7 bones between the foot and the leg)
tax/o	order; coordination
tel/o	complete
tele/o	distant
ten/o	tendon
tendin/o	tendon
-tension	pressure
terat/o	monster; malformed fetus
test/o	testis (testicle)
tetra-	four

MEDICAL WORD PARTS—ENGLISH
(Continued)

COMBINING FORM, SUFFIX, OR PREFIX	MEANING
thalam/o	thalamus
thalass/o	sea
the/o	put; place
thec/o	sheath
thel/o	nipple
therapeut/o	treatment
-therapy	treatment
therm/o	heat
thorac/o	chest
-thorax	chest; pleural cavity
thromb/o	clot
thym/o	thymus gland
-thymia	mind (condition of)
-thymic	pertaining to mind
thyr/o	thyroid gland; shield
thyroid/o	thyroid gland
tibi/o	tibia (shin bone)
-tic	pertaining to
toc/o	labor; birth
-tocia	labor; birth (condition of)
-tocin	labor; birth (a substance for)
tom/o	to cut
-tome	instrument to cut
-tomy	process of cutting
ton/o	tension
tone/o	to stretch
tonsill/o	tonsil
top/o	place; position; location
-tory	pertaining to
tox/o	poison
toxic/o	poison
trache/o	trachea (windpipe)
trans-	across; through
-tresia	opening
tri-	three
trich/o	hair

MEDICAL WORD PARTS—ENGLISH
(Continued)

COMBINING FORM, SUFFIX, OR PREFIX	MEANING
trigon/o	trigone (area within the bladder)
-tripsy	crushing
troph/o	nourishment; development
-trophy	nourishment; development (condition of)
-tropia	to turn
-tropic	pertaining to stimulating
-tropin	stimulate; act on
tympan/o	tympanic membrane (eardrum); middle ear
-type	classification; picture
-ule	little; small
uln/o	ulna (medial lower arm bone)
ultra-	beyond; excess
-um	structure; tissue; thing
umbilic/o	umbilicus (navel)
ungu/o	nail
uni-	one
ur/o	urine; urinary tract
ureter/o	ureter
urethr/o	urethra
-uria	urination; condition of urine
urin/o	urine
-us	structure; thing
uter/o	uterus (womb)
uve/o	uvea, vascular layer of eye (iris, choroid, ciliary body)
uvul/o	uvula
vag/o	vagus nerve
vagin/o	vagina
valv/o	valve
valvul/o	valve
varic/o	varicose veins
vas/o	vessel; duct; vas deferens

MEDICAL WORD PARTS—ENGLISH
(Continued)

COMBINING FORM, SUFFIX, OR PREFIX	MEANING
vascul/o	vessel (blood)
ven/o, ven/i	vein
vener/o	venereal (sexual contact)
ventr/o	belly side of body
ventricul/o	ventricle (of heart or brain)
venul/o	venule (small vein)
-verse	to turn
-version	to turn
vertebr/o	vertebra (backbone)
vesic/o	urinary bladder
vesicul/o	seminal vesicle
vestibul/o	vestibule of the inner ear
viscer/o	internal organs
vit/o	life
vitr/o	vitreous body (of the eye)
vitre/o	glass
viv/o	life
vol/o	to roll
vulv/o	vulva (female external genitalia)
xanth/o	yellow
xen/o	stranger
xer/o	dry
xiph/o	sword
-y	condition; process
zo/o	animal life

ENGLISH—MEDICAL WORD PARTS

MEANING	COMBINING FORM, SUFFIX, OR PREFIX
abdomen	abdomin/o (*use with* -al, -centesis)
	celi/o (*use with* -ac)
	lapar/o (*use with* -scope, -scopy, -tomy)
abdominal wall	lapar/o
abnormal	dys-
	par-
	para-
abnormal condition	-iasis
	-osis
above	epi-
	hyper-
	supra-
acetabulum	acetabul/o
acetones	ket/o
	keton/o
acid	oxy-
acromion	acromi/o
across	trans-
action	-praxia
act on	-tropin
adrenal glands	adren/o
	adrenal/o
after	post-
again	ana-, re-
against	anti-
	contra-
air	aer/o
	pneum/o
	pneumon/o
air sac	alveol/o
albumin	albumin/o
all	pan-
along the side of	para-
alveolus	alveol/o

ENGLISH—MEDICAL WORD PARTS
(Continued)

MEANING	COMBINING FORM, SUFFIX, OR PREFIX
anew	ana-
amnion	amni/o
aneurysm	aneurysm/o
angle	goni/o
animal life	zo/o
animal starch	glycogen/o
ankle	tars/o
antrum (of stomach)	antr/o
anus	an/o
anus and rectum	proct/o
anxiety	anxi/o
apart	ana-
apart from	para-
appendix	append/o (*use with* -ectomy)
	appendic/o (*use with* -itis)
appetite	-orexia
arm	brachi/o
arm bone, lower, lateral	radi/o
arm bone, lower, medial	uln/o
arm bone, upper	humer/o
armpit	axill/o
arteriole	arteriol/o
artery	arter/o
	arteri/o
articulate (speak distinctly)	-arthria
asbestos	asbest/o
assemble	-agon
atrium	atri/o
attraction for	-phil
	-philia
attraction to	phil/o

ENGLISH—MEDICAL WORD PARTS
(Continued)

MEANING	COMBINING FORM, SUFFIX, OR PREFIX
auditory tube	salping/o
away from	ab-
	apo-
	ex-
	exo-
back	re-
	retro-
back, lower	lumb/o
back portion of body	dorsi-
	dors/o
	poster/o
backbone	spin/o (*use with* -al)
	spondyl/o (*use with* -itis, -listhesis, -osis, -pathy)
	vertebr/o (*use with* -al)
backward	ana-
	retro-
bacteria	bacteri/o
bacterium (berry-shaped)	-coccus (-cocci, *pl.*)
bacilli (rod-shaped bacteria)	bacill/o
bad	cac/o
	dys-
	mal-
barrier	claustr/o
base (not acidic)	bas/o
bear, to	-para
	-parous
	-phoria
	phor/o
before	ante-
	pre-
	pro-
	pros-

ENGLISH—MEDICAL WORD PARTS
(Continued)

MEANING	COMBINING FORM, SUFFIX, OR PREFIX
beginning	-arche
behind	post-
	poster/o
	retro-
belly	celi/o
belly side of body	ventr/o
below, beneath	hypo-
	infra-
	sub-
bend, to	flex/o
bent	scoli/o
beside	para-
between	inter-
beyond	hyper-
	meta-
	ultra-
bile	bil/i
	chol/e
bile vessel	cholangi/o
bilirubin	bilirubin/o
bind	-desis
	nect/o
birth	nat/i
	-partum
	toc/o
	-tocia
birth, substance for	-tocin
births, live	-para
black	anthrac/o
	melan/o
bladder (urinary)	cyst/o (*use with* -ic, -itis, -cele, -gram, -scopy, -stomy, -tomy)
	vesic/o (*use with* -al)

ENGLISH—MEDICAL WORD PARTS
(Continued)

MEANING	COMBINING FORM, SUFFIX, OR PREFIX
blood	hem/o (*use with* -dialysis, -globin, -lysis, -philia, -ptysis, -rrhage, -stasis, -stat)
	hemat/o (*use with* -crit, -emesis, -logist, -logy, -oma, -poiesis, -uria)
blood condition	-emia
	-emic
blood vessel	angi/o (*use with* -ectomy, -genesis, -gram, -graphy, -oma, -plasty, -spasm)
	vas/o (*use with* -constriction, -dilation, -motor)
	vascul/o (*use with* -ar, -itis)
blue	cyan/o
body	corpor/o
	somat/o
	-some
bone	oste/o
bone condition	-ostosis
bone marrow	myel/o
brain	encephal/o
branching	furc/o
break	-clasis
	-clast
breakdown	-lysis
breast	mamm/o (*use with* -ary, -gram, -graphy, -plasty)
	mast/o (*use with* -algia, -dynia, -ectomy, -itis)

ENGLISH—MEDICAL WORD PARTS
(Continued)

MEANING	COMBINING FORM, SUFFIX, OR PREFIX
breastbone	stern/o
breathe	spir/o
breathing	-pnea
bring forth	-para
	-parous
bronchial tube	bronch/o
(bronchus)	bronchi/o
bronchiole	bronchiol/o
bunion	bunion/o
burn	caus/o
	cauter/o
bursa	burs/o
bursting forth	-rrhage
	-rrhagia
calcaneus	calcane/o
calcium	calc/o
	calci/o
calculus	lith/o
calyx	cali/o
	calic/o
cancerous	carcin/o
capillary	capillar/o
carbon dioxide	capn/o
	-capnia
care for, to	comi/o
carry	duct/o
	-phoresis
	-phoria
carrying	-ferent
cartilage	chondr/o
cast; throw	bol/o
cause	eti/o
cecum	cec/o
cell	cyt/o
	-cyte

ENGLISH—MEDICAL WORD PARTS
(Continued)

MEANING	COMBINING FORM, SUFFIX, OR PREFIX
cells, condition of	-cytosis
cerebellum	cerebell/o
cerebrum	cerebr/o
cerumen	cerumin/o
cervix	cervic/o
change	meta-
cheek	bucc/o
chemical	chem/o
chest	pector/o
	steth/o
	thorac/o
	-thorax
child	ped/o
childbirth	obstetr/o
chin	ment/o
cholesterol	cholesterol/o
chorion	chori/o
	chorion/o
choroid layer (of the eye)	choroid/o
ciliary body (of the eye)	cycl/o
circle *or* cycle	cycl/o
clavicle (collar bone)	clavicul/o
clot	thromb/o
clumping	agglutin/o
clusters	staphyl/o
coagulation	coagul/o
coal dust	anthrac/o
coccyx	coccyg/o
cochlea	cochle/o
cold	cry/o
collar bone	clavicul/o
colon	col/o (*use with* -ectomy, -itis, -pexy, -stomy)
	colon/o (*use with* -ic, -pathy, -scope, -scopy)

ENGLISH—MEDICAL WORD PARTS
(Continued)

MEANING	COMBINING FORM, SUFFIX, OR PREFIX
color	chrom/o
come together	-fusion
common bile duct	choledoch/o
complete	dia-
	tel/o
condition	-ation
	-ema
	-esis
	-ia
	-ism
	-itus
	-sis
	-y
condition, abnormal	-iasis
	-osis
connect	nect/o
connective tissue	sarc/o
constant	home/o
control	-stasis, -stat
contraction	-stalsis
contraction of muscles, sudden	-spasm
coordination	tax/o
copy	-mimetic
cornea (of the eye)	corne/o
	kerat/o
cortex	cortic/o
cotton dust	byssin/o
crooked	scoli/o
crushing	-tripsy
curve	lord/o
cut	cis/o
	sect/o, -section
	tom/o
cut off	syncop/o

ENGLISH—MEDICAL WORD PARTS
(Continued)

MEANING	COMBINING FORM, SUFFIX, OR PREFIX
cutting, process of	-tomy
cycle	cycl/o
cyst (sac of fluid)	cyst/o
dance	chore/o
dark	phe/o
darkness	scot/o
dawn-colored	eosin/o
death	leth/o
	mort/o, -mortem
	necr/o
defecation	-chezia
deficiency	-penia
deficient	hypo-
derived from	-oid
destroying	-lytic
destruction	-lysis
development	plas/o
	-plasia
	troph/o
	-trophy
diaphragm	phren/o
difficult	dys-
digestion	-pepsia
dilation	-ectasia
	-ectasis
dim	ambly/o
discharge	-rrhea
disease	nos/o
	path/o
	-pathy
distant	dist/o
	tele/o
distinct	idi/o
double	dipl/o

ENGLISH—MEDICAL WORD PARTS
(Continued)

MEANING	COMBINING FORM, SUFFIX, OR PREFIX
down	cata-
	de-
drooping	-ptosis
drug	chem/o
	pharmac/o
	pharmaceut/o
dry	ichthy/o
	xer/o
drying	desicc/o
duct	vas/o
dull	ambly/o
duodenum	duoden/o
dura mater	dur/o
dusky	phe/o
dust	coni/o
ear	aur/o (*use with* -al, -icle)
	auricul/o (*use with* -ar)
	ot/o (*use with* -algia, -ic, -itis, -logy, -mycosis, -rrhea, -sclerosis, -scope, -scopy)
ear, condition of	-otia
eardrum	myring/o (*use with* -ectomy, -itis, -tomy)
	tympan/o (*use with* -ic, -metry, -plasty)
eat	phag/o
	-phage
eating	-phagia
egg cell	o/o
	ov/o
	ovul/o
elbow	olecran/o
electricity	electr/o
elimination of wastes	-chezia

MEANING	COMBINING FORM, SUFFIX, OR PREFIX
embryonic	-blast
enlargement	-megaly
enzyme	-ase
epididymis	epididym/o
epiglottis	epiglott/o
equal	is/o
esophagus	esophag/o
eustachian tube	salping/o
excess	ultra-
excessive	hyper-
excision	-ectomy
expansion	-ectasia
	-ectasis
extreme	pol/o
extreme point	acr/o
extremities	acr/o
eye	ocul/o (*use with* -ar, -facial, -motor)
	ophthalm/o (*use with* -ia, -ic, -logist, -logy, -pathy, -plasty, -plegia, -scope, -scopy)
	opt/o (*use with* -ic, -metrist)
	optic/o (*use with* -al, -ian)
eyelid	blephar/o (*use with* -chalasis, -itis, -plasty, -plegia, -ptosis, -tomy)
	palpebr/o (*use with* -al)
face	faci/o
faint	syncop/o
falling	-ptosis
fallopian tube	salping/o
	-salpinx
false	pseudo-
far	dist/o
fascia	fasci/o

ENGLISH—MEDICAL WORD PARTS
(Continued)

MEANING	COMBINING FORM, SUFFIX, OR PREFIX
fast	tachy-
fat	adip/o (*use with* -ose, -osis)
	lip/o (*use with* -ase, -cyte, -genesis, -oid, -oma)
	steat/o (*use with* -oma, -rrhea)
fear	phob/o
	-phobia
feeling	esthesi/o
	-phoria
female	estr/o (*use with* -gen, -genic)
	gynec/o (*use with* -logist, -logy, -mastia)
femur	femor/o
fever	pyr/o
	pyret/o
	pyrex/o
fiber	fibr/o
fibrous connective tissue	fibros/o
fibula	fibul/o (*use with* -ar)
	perone/o (*use with* -al)
finger and toe bones	phalang/o
fingers	dactyl/o
fire	pyr/o
first	prot/o
fixation	-pexy
flat plate	-elasma
flesh	sarc/o
flow	-rrhea
fluid collection	-oma
flushed	erythem/o
foot	pod/o

ENGLISH—MEDICAL WORD PARTS
(Continued)

MEANING	COMBINING FORM, SUFFIX, OR PREFIX
foot bones	metatars/o
forking	furc/o
form	morph/o
formation	plas/o
	-plasia
	-plasm
	-poiesis
forming	-genesis
forward	ante-, pro-, pros-
four	quadri-
front	anter/o
full of	-ose
fungus	fung/i (*use with* -cide, -oid, -ous, -stasis)
	myc/o (*use with* -logist, -logy, -osis, -tic)
gall	bil/i (*use with* -ary)
	chol/e (*use with* -lithiasis)
gallbladder	cholecyst/o
ganglion	gangli/o
	ganglion/o
gas	pneum/o
	pneumon/o
gather	-agon
genetic change	mut/a
	mutagen/o
give, to	-dote
given, what is	-dote
gland	aden/o
glans penis	balan/o
glass	silic/o
	vitre/o
glial cells	gli/o
globe-shaped	spher/o

ENGLISH—MEDICAL WORD PARTS
(Continued)

MEANING	COMBINING FORM, SUFFIX, OR PREFIX
glomerulus	glomerul/o
glucose	gluc/o
	glyc/o
	glycos/o
glue	coll/a
	gli/o
glycogen	glycogen/o
go, to	-grade
good	eu-
granule(s)	granul/o
gray	glauc/o
gray matter	poli/o
green	chlor/o
groin	inguin/o
grow	-physis
growth	-plasia
gum	gingiv/o
habit	-hexia
hair	pil/o
	trich/o
half	hemi-
	semi-
hallucination	hallucin/o
hand	chir/o
hand bones	metacarp/o
hang, to	pend/o
hard	kerat/o
	scirrh/o
hardening	-sclerosis
	scler/o
head	cephal/o
hearing	acous/o
	audi/o
	audit/o
	-acusis
	-cusis

ENGLISH—MEDICAL WORD PARTS
(Continued)

MEANING	COMBINING FORM, SUFFIX, OR PREFIX
heart	cardi/o (*use with* -ac, -graphy, -logy, -logist, -megaly, -pathy, -vascular)
	coron/o (*use with* -ary)
heart muscle	myocardi/o
heat	cauter/o
	therm/o
heavy	pachy-
heel bone	calcane/o
hemoglobin	hemoglobin/o
hernia	-cele
	herni/o
hidden	crypt/o
hip region	pelv/i, pelv/o
holding back	isch/o
hormone	hormon/o
	-one
horn-like	kerat/o
horse	equin/o
humerus	humer/o
humpback	kyph/o
hydrochloric acid	chlorhydr/o
ileum	ile/o
ilium	ili/o
immature cell	-blast
immature tumor (cells)	-blastoma
immune	immun/o
in, into, within	em-
	en-
	endo-
	in-, intra-
	ir-
in due measure	emmetr/o

ENGLISH—MEDICAL WORD PARTS
(Continued)

MEANING	COMBINING FORM, SUFFIX, OR PREFIX
in front of	pre-
incomplete	atel/o
increase in cell numbers (blood cells)	-cytosis
individual	idi/o
infection	seps/o
inferior to	infra-
inflammation	-itis
instrument for recording	-graph
instrument for visual examination	-scope
instrument to cut	-tome
insulin	insulin/o
internal organs	splanchn/o
	viscer/o
intestine, large	col/o
intestine, small	enter/o
iodine	iod/o
ion	ion/o
iris	ir/o
	irid/o
iron	sider/o
irregular	poikil/o
irrigation	-clysis
ischium	ischi/o
itching	prurit/o
jaw, lower	mandibul/o
	submaxill/o
jaw, upper	maxill/o
joint	arthr/o
	articul/o
ketones	ket/o
	keton/o

ENGLISH—MEDICAL WORD PARTS
(Continued)

MEANING	COMBINING FORM, SUFFIX, OR PREFIX
kidney	nephr/o (*use with* -algia, -ectomy, -ic, -itis, -lith, -megaly, -oma, -osis, -pathy, -ptosis, -sclerosis, -stomy, -tomy)
	ren/o (*use with* -al, -gram, -vascular)
killing	-cidal
	-cide
knowledge	gnos/o, gno/o
labor	-partum
	toc/o
	-tocia
labor, substance for	-tocin
lack of	de-
lack of strength	-asthenia
lacrimal duct	dacry/o
	lacrim/o
lacrimal sac	dacryocyst/o
lamina	lamin/o
large	macro-
	mega-
larynx	laryng/o
lead	duct/o
lens of eye	phac/o
	phak/o
less	de-
	mi/o
less than normal	hypo-
life	bi/o
	vit/o
	viv/o
ligament	ligament/o
	syndesm/o

ENGLISH—MEDICAL WORD PARTS
(Continued)

MEANING	COMBINING FORM, SUFFIX, OR PREFIX
like	phil/o
lip	cheil/o
	labi/o
lipid	lip/o
little	-ole
	-ule
liver	hepat/o
lobe	lob/o
location	top/o
loin	lumb/o
loosening	-lysis
love	phil/o
luminous	fluor/o
lung	pneum/o (*use with* -coccus, -coniosis, -thorax)
	pneumon/o (*use with* -ectomy, -ia, -ic, -itis, -lysis)
	pulmon/o (*use with* -ary)
lymph	lymph/o
lymph gland	lymphaden/o
lymph vessel	lymphangi/o
make, to	-fication
male	andr/o
malformed fetus	terat/o
malleolus	malleol/o
mandible	mandibul/o
	submaxill/o
many	multi-
	ple/o
	poly-
marketplace	agora-
marrow	medull/o
mass	-oma

ENGLISH—MEDICAL WORD PARTS
(Continued)

MEANING	COMBINING FORM, SUFFIX, OR PREFIX
mastoid process	mastoid/o
maxilla	maxill/o
meal	cib/o
	-prandial
measure	-meter
	metr/o
meatus	meat/o
mediastinum	mediastin/o
medulla oblongata	medull/o
meninges	mening/o
	meningi/o
menstruation; menses	men/o
metacarpals	metacarp/o
metatarsals	metatars/o
middle	medi/o
	medull/o
	meso-
middle ear	tympan/o
midwife	obstetr/o
milk	galact/o
	lact/o
mimic	-mimetic
mind	ment/o
	phren/o
	psych/o
	-thymia
	-thymic
mixture	cras/o
monster	terat/o
mood	-thymia
	-thymic
more	ple/o
mouth	or/o (*use with* -al)
	stomat/o (*use with* -itis)
	-stomia

ENGLISH—MEDICAL WORD PARTS
(Continued)

MEANING	COMBINING FORM, SUFFIX, OR PREFIX
movement	cine/o
	kines/o
	kinesi/o
	-kinesia
	-kinesis
	-motor
much	poly-
mucous membrane	mucos/o
mucus	muc/o
	myx/o
muscle	muscul/o (*use with* -ar, -skeletal)
	my/o (*use with* -algia, -ectomy, -oma, -neural, -pathy, -rrhaphy, -therapy)
	myos/o (*use with* -in, -itis)
muscle, heart	myocardi/o
muscle, smooth (visceral)	leiomy/o
muscle, striated (skeletal)	rhabdomy/o
muscle tumor	myom/o
muzzle	phim/o
nail	onych/o
	ungu/o
narrowing	-constriction
	sten/o
	-stenosis
nature	physi/o
navel	omphal/o
	umbilic/o
neck	cervic/o
neither	neutr/o

ENGLISH—MEDICAL WORD PARTS
(Continued)

MEANING	COMBINING FORM, SUFFIX, OR PREFIX
nerve	neur/o
nerve root	radicul/o
nest	nid/o
new	neo-
network	reticul/o
network of nerves	plex/o
neutral	neutr/o
neutrophil	neutr/o
night	noct/o
	nyct/o
nipple	thel/o
nipple-like	papill/o
nitrogen	azot/o
nitrogen compound	-amine
no, not	a-
	an-
none	nulli-
normal	eu-
nose	nas/o (*use with* -al)
	rhin/o (*use with* -itis, -rrhea, -plasty)
nourishment	troph/o
	-trophy
nucleus	kary/o
	nucle/o
nucleus (collection of nerve cells in the brain)	kern-
numbness	narc/o
obscure	-opaque
obsessive preoccupation	-mania
off	apo-
old age	ger/o, geront/o
	presby/o
olecranon (elbow)	olecran/o

ENGLISH—MEDICAL WORD PARTS
(Continued)

MEANING	COMBINING FORM, SUFFIX, OR PREFIX
on	epi-
one	mon/o
	mono-
	uni-
one's own	aut/o
	auto-
one who	-er
	-or
opening	-tresia
opening, new	-stomy
opposite	contra-
optic disc (disk)	papill/o
orange-yellow	cirrh/o
order	norm/o
	tax/o
organs, internal	viscer/o
ossicle	ossicul/o
other	all/o
other than	par-
out, outside	ec-
	ex-
	exo-
	extra-
outer region	cortic/o
ovary	oophor/o (*use with* -itis, -ectomy, -pexy)
	ovari/o (*use with* -an)
own	aut-
oxygen	ox/o
	-oxia
pain	-algia (*use with* arthr/o, cephal/o, gastr/o, mast/o, my/o, neur/o, ot/o)
	-dynia (*use with* coccyg/o, pleur/o)
	odyn/o

ENGLISH—MEDICAL WORD PARTS
(Continued)

MEANING	COMBINING FORM, SUFFIX, OR PREFIX
pain, excessive	-agra
pain, sensitivity to	-algesia
	algesi/o
painful	dys-
palate	palat/o
palsy	-plegia
	-plegic
pancreas	pancreat/o
paralysis	-plegia
	-plegic
paralysis, slight	-paresis
patella	patell/a (*use with* -pexy)
	patell/o (*use with* -ar, -ectomy, -femoral)
pelvis	pelv/i
	pelv/o
penis	balan/o
	pen/o
	phall/o
people	dem/o
perineum	perine/o
peritoneum	peritone/o
pertaining to	-ac (*as in* cardiac)
	-al (*as in* inguinal)
	-an (*as in* ovarian)
	-ar (*as in* palmar)
	-ary (*as in* papillary)
	-eal (*as in* pharyngeal)
	-iac (*as in* hypochondriac)
	-ic (*as in* nucleic)
	-ical (*as in* psychological)
	-ile (*as in* penile)
	-ine (*as in* equine)
	-ior (*as in* superior)
	-ose (*as in* adipose)
	-ous (*as in* mucous)
	-tic (*as in* necrotic)
	-tory (*as in* secretory)

ENGLISH—MEDICAL WORD PARTS
(Continued)

MEANING	COMBINING FORM, SUFFIX, OR PREFIX
phalanges	phalang/o
pharynx (throat)	pharyng/o
phrase	-lexia
physician	iatr/o
pineal gland	pineal/o
pituitary gland	hypophys/o
	pituit/o
	pituitar/o
place	-stasis
	the/o
	top/o
plant	phyt/o
	-phyte
plaque	ather/o
	-plakia
pleura	pleur/o
pleural cavity	-thorax
plexus	plex/o
poison	tox/o
	toxic/o
pole	styl/o
polyp	polyp/o
pons	pont/o
pores, condition of	-porosis
position	top/o
potassium	kal/i
pour	chym/o
	-fusion
pregnancy	-cyesis
	gest/o
	gester/o
	gravid/o
	-gravida
	obstetr/o

ENGLISH—MEDICAL WORD PARTS
(Continued)

MEANING	COMBINING FORM, SUFFIX, OR PREFIX
pressure	bar/o
	-tension
process	-ation
	-ion
	-ism
	-y
produced by *or* in	-genic
producing	-gen
	-genesis
prolapse	-ptosis
prostate gland	prostat/o
protection	immun/o
	-phylaxis
protein	albumin/o
	-globin
	-globulin
	prote/o
pubis	pub/o
pulse	sphygm/o
	-sphyxia
puncture to remove fluid	-centesis
pupil	cor/o
	core/o
	pupill/o
pus	py/o, purul/o
put	the/o
put in place	-pexy
pyloric sphincter, pylorus	pylor/o
radioactivity	radi/o
radius (lower arm bone)	radi/o
rapid	oxy-
rash	exanthemat/o

ENGLISH—MEDICAL WORD PARTS
(Continued)

MEANING	COMBINING FORM, SUFFIX, OR PREFIX
rays	radi/o
record	-gram
recording, process of	-graphy
rectum	rect/o
recurring	cycl/o
red	eosin/o
	erythr/o
redness	erythem/o
	erythemat/o
reduce	-lytic
relaxation	-chalasia, -chalasis
removal	-apheresis
	-ectomy
	-pheresis
renal pelvis	pyel/o
repair	-plasty
resembling	-form
	-oid
retina	retin/o
rib	cost/o
roll, to	vol/o
rosy	eosin/o
round	spher/o
rule	norm/o
run	-drome
rupture	-rrhexis
sac, small	alveol/o
	follicul/o
sac of fluid	cyst/o
sacrum	sacr/o
safe	immun/o
sag, to	-ptosis
saliva	sial/o
salivary gland	sialaden/o
same	ipsi-
	is/o

ENGLISH—MEDICAL WORD PARTS
(Continued)

MEANING	COMBINING FORM, SUFFIX, OR PREFIX
sameness	home/o
scaly	ichthy/o
scanty	olig/o
sclera	scler/o
scrotum	scrot/o
sea	thalass/o
sebum	seb/o
	sebace/o
	steat/o
secrete	crin/o
	-crine
seed	gon/o
	semin/i
seizure	-lepsy
seizing, taking hold of (pertaining to)	-leptic
self	aut/o
	auto-
semen	semin/i
seminal vesicle	vesicul/o
send, sending	-mission
sensation (nervous)	-esthesia
separate, to	-crit
	-crine
	-lytic
separation	-lysis
set, to	-stitial
severe	acu/o
sex glands	gonad/o
sexual intercourse	-pareunia
shape	-form
	morph/o
sharp	acu/o
	oxy-
sheath	thec/o
shield	thyr/o
shin bone	tibi/o
shine	-lucent

ENGLISH—MEDICAL WORD PARTS
(Continued)

MEANING	COMBINING FORM, SUFFIX, OR PREFIX
short	brachy-
shoulder	om/o
side	later/o
sieve	ethm/o
sigmoid colon	sigmoid/o
single	mon/o
sinus	sinus/o
skin	cutane/o (*use with* -ous)
	derm/o (*use with* -al)
	-derma (*use with* erythr/o, leuk/o)
	dermat/o (*use with* -itis, -logist, -logy, -osis)
	epitheli/o (*use with* -al, -lysis, -oid, -oma, -um)
skull	crani/o
sleep	hypn/o
	somn/o
	-somnia
sleep, deep	comat/o
slender	lept/o
slide, to	lux/o
sliding, condition of	-lapse
slipping	-listhesis
slow	brady-
small	-icle
	micro-
	-ole
	-ule
small intestine	enter/o
smaller	mi/o
smell	-osmia
sodium	natr/o
soft	medull/o
softening	-malacia
sole (of the foot)	plant/o

ENGLISH—MEDICAL WORD PARTS
(Continued)

MEANING	COMBINING FORM, SUFFIX, OR PREFIX
solution	-sol
sound	echo-
	phon/o
	-phonia
	son/o
spark	scint/i
specialist	-ist
speech	phas/o
	-phasia
sperm cells (spermatozoa)	sperm/o
	spermat/o
spinal column (spine)	spin/o
	rachi/o
	vertebr/o
spinal cord	myel/o
spiny	acanth/o
spitting	-ptysis
spleen	splen/o
split	-fida
	schiz/o
split	-schisis
stake (pole)	styl/o
stapes	staped/o
starch	amyl/o
state of	-sis
	-hexia
steal	klept/o
sternum	stern/o
steroid	ster/o
sticking together	agglutin/o
stiff	ankyl/o
stimulate	-tropin
	-tropic
stomach	gastr/o
stone	lith/o
stop	-suppression

ENGLISH—MEDICAL WORD PARTS
(Continued)

MEANING	COMBINING FORM, SUFFIX, OR PREFIX
stopping	-stasis
	-static
straight	orth/o
stranger	xen/o
strength	-sthenia
stretch	tone/o
stretching	-ectasia
	-ectasis
stricture	-stenosis
structure	-ium
	-plasm
	-um, -us
structure, solid	ster/o
study of	log/o
	-logy
stupor	narc/o
substance	-in
	-ine
substance that forms	-poietin
sudden	acu/o
	oxysm/o
sugar	gluc/o
	glyc/o
	glycos/o
	-ose
surgical repair	-plasty
surrounding	peri-
suture	-rrhaphy
swallow	phag/o
swallowing	-phagia
swayback	lord/o
sweat	diaphor/o (*use with* -esis)
	hidr/o (*use with* -osis)
sword	xiph/o
synovia (fluid)	synov/o
synovial membrane	synov/o

ENGLISH—MEDICAL WORD PARTS
(Continued)

MEANING	COMBINING FORM, SUFFIX, OR PREFIX
tail	caud/o
tailbone	coccyg/o
tear	dacry/o (*use with* -genic, -rrhea)
	lacrim/o (*use with* -al, -ation)
tearing (cutting)	-spadia
tear gland	dacryoaden/o
tear sac	dacryocyst/o
temperament	cras/o
tendon	ten/o
	tend/o
	tendin/o
tension	ton/o
testis	orch/o (*use with* -itis)
	orchi/o (*use with* -algia, -dynia, -ectomy, -pathy, -pexy, -tomy)
	orchid/o (*use with* -ectomy, -pexy, -plasty, -ptosis, -tomy)
	test/o (*use with* -sterone)
thick	pachy-
thigh bone	femor/o
thin	lept/o
thing	-um
	-us
thing that produces	-gen
thirst	dips/o
thorny	acanth/o
three	tri-
throat	pharyng/o
through	dia-
	per-
	trans-
throw, to	bol/o

ENGLISH—MEDICAL WORD PARTS
(Continued)

MEANING	COMBINING FORM, SUFFIX, OR PREFIX
thymus gland	thym/o
thyroid gland	thyr/o
	thyroid/o
tibia	tibi/o
tie	nect/o
tie together	-desis
tightening	-stenosis
time	chron/o
tissue	hist/o
	histi/o
	-ium
	-um
toes	dactyl/o
together	con-
	sym-
	syn-
tongue	gloss/o (*use with* -al, -dynia, -plasty, -plegia, -rrhaphy, -spasm, -tomy)
	lingu/o (*use with* -al)
tonsil	tonsill/o
tooth	dent/i
	odont/o
top	acr/o
toward	ad-
	af-
	-ad
trachea	trache/o
transmission	-phoresis
treatment	iatr/o
	therapeut/o
	-therapy
trigone	trigon/o
tube	syring/o

ENGLISH—MEDICAL WORD PARTS
(Continued)

MEANING	COMBINING FORM, SUFFIX, OR PREFIX
tumor	-oma
	onc/o
turn	-tropia
	-verse
	-version
twisted chains	strept/o
two	bi-
tympanic membrane	myring/o
	tympan/o
ulcer	aphth/o
ulna	uln/o
umbilicus, navel	omphal/o (*use with* -cele, -ectomy, -rrhagia, -rrhexis)
	umbilic/o (*use with* -al)
unchanging	home/o
under	hypo-
unequal	anis/o
unknown	idi/o
up	ana-
upon	epi-
urea	azot/o
ureter	ureter/o
urethra	urethr/o
urinary bladder	cyst/o (*use with* -cele, -ectomy, -itis, -pexy, -plasty, -plegia, -scope, -scopy, -stomy, -tomy)
	vesic/o (*use with* -al)
urinary tract	ur/o
urination	-uria
urine	ur/o
	-uria
	urin/o

ENGLISH—MEDICAL WORD PARTS
(Continued)

MEANING	COMBINING FORM, SUFFIX, OR PREFIX
uterus	hyster/o (*use with* -ectomy, -graphy, -gram, -tomy)
	metr/o (*use with* -rrhagia, -rrhea, -rrhexis)
	metri/o (*use with* -osis)
	uter/o (*use with* -ine)
uvea	uve/o
uvula	uvul/o (*use with* -ar, -itis, -ptosis)
	staphyl/o (*use with* -ectomy, -plasty, -tomy)
vagina	colp/o (*use with* -pexy, -plasty, -scope, -scopy, -tomy)
	vagin/o (*use with* -al, -itis)
vagus nerve	vag/o
valve	valv/o
	valvul/o
varicose veins	varic/o
varied	poikil/o
	ple/o
vas deferens	vas/o
vein	phleb/o (*use with* -ectomy, -itis, -tomy)
	ven/o (*use with* -ous, -gram)
	ven/i (*use with* -puncture)
vein, small	venul/o
venereal	vener/o
ventricle	ventricul/o

ENGLISH—MEDICAL WORD PARTS
(Continued)

MEANING	COMBINING FORM, SUFFIX, OR PREFIX
vertebra	rachi/o (*use with* -itis, -tomy)
	spondyl/o (*use with* -itis, -listhesis, -osis, -pathy)
	vertebr/o (*use with* -al)
vessel	angi/o (*use with* -ectomy, -genesis, -gram, -graphy, -oma, -plasty, -spasm)
	vas/o (*use with* -constriction, -dilation, -motor)
	vascul/o (*use with* -ar, -itis)
view of	-opsy
viscera	splanchn/o
vision	-opia
	-opsia
	opt/o
	optic/o
visual examination	-scopy
vitreous body	vitr/o
voice	phon/o
	-phonia
voice box	laryng/o
vomiting	-emesis
vulva	episi/o (*use with* -tomy)
	vulv/o (*use with* -ar)
wander	ion/o
washing	-clysis
wasting away	-phthisis
water	aque/o
	hydr/o
watery flow	rheumat/o
weakness	-paresis
wedge	sphen/o

ENGLISH—MEDICAL WORD PARTS
(Continued)

MEANING	COMBINING FORM, SUFFIX, OR PREFIX
weight	bar/o
white	alb/o
	albin/o
	leuk/o
wide	mydr/o
widening	-dilation
	-ectasia
	-ectasis
	-eurysm
windpipe	trache/o
with	con-
	sym-
	syn-
within	en-, end-
	endo-
	intra-
woman	gynec/o
womb	hyster/o
	metr/o
	metri/o
	uter/o
word	-lexia
work	erg/o
wrinkle	rhytid/o
wrist bone	carp/o
x-rays	radi/o
yellow	lute/o
	jaund/o
	xanth/o

Abbreviations*

Many of these abbreviations may appear with or without periods and with either a capital or a lowercase first letter. (Latin abbreviations are spelled out in *italics* in parentheses.)

A, B, AB, O	blood types; may have subscript numbers
A2, A$_2$	aortic valve closure (a heart sound)
@	at
ā	before
AAA	abdominal aortic aneurysm
AAL	anterior axillary line
AB, ab	abortion
Ab	antibody
ABCDE	asymmetry (of shape), border (irregularity), color (variation with one lesion), diameter (greater than 6 mm), evolution (change)—characteristics associated with melanoma
abd	abdomen; abduction
ABGs	arterial blood gases
AC	acromioclavicular (joint)
ac, a.c.	before meals (*ante cibum*)
ACE	angiotensin-converting enzyme (ACE inhibitors treat hypertension)
ACh	acetylcholine (a neurotransmitter)
ACL	anterior cruciate ligament (of knee)
ACLS	advanced cardiac life support

---

*From Chabner DE: The Language of Medicine, 9th ed. Philadelphia, Saunders, 2011.

Abbreviations (Continued)

ACS	acute coronary syndrome(s)
ACTH	adrenocorticotropic hormone (secreted by the anterior pituitary gland)
AD	Alzheimer disease
A.D.	right ear (*auris dextra*); better to specify "right ear" rather than abbreviating)
ad lib.	as desired (*ad libitum*, "freely")
ADD	attention deficit disorder
add	adduction
ADH	antidiuretic hormone; vasopressin (secreted by the posterior pituitary gland)
ADHD	attention-deficit hyperactivity disorder
ADL	activities of daily living
ADT	admission, discharge, transfer
AED	automated external defibrillator
AF	atrial fibrillation
AFB	acid-fast bacillus/bacilli—the TB organism
AFO	ankle-foot orthosis (device for stabilization)
AFP	alpha-fetoprotein
Ag	silver (*argentum*)
AHF	antihemophilic factor (same as coagulation factor XIII)
AICD	automatic implantable cardioverter-defibrillator
AIDS	acquired immunodeficiency syndrome
AIHA	autoimmune hemolytic anemia
AKA	above-knee amputation
alb	albumin (protein)
alk phos	alkaline phosphatase (elevated in liver disease)
ALL	acute lymphocytic leukemia
ALS	amyotrophic lateral sclerosis (Lou Gehrig disease)

Abbreviations (Continued)

ALT	alanine aminotransferase (elevated in liver and heart disease); formerly called serum glutamic-pyruvic transaminase (SGPT)
AM, a.m., AM	in the morning *or* before noon (*ante meridiem*)
AMA	against medical advice; American Medical Association
amb	ambulate, ambulatory (walking)
AMD	age-related macular degeneration
AMI	acute myocardial infarction
AML	acute myelocytic/myelogenous leukemia
ANA	antinuclear antibody
ANC	absolute neutrophil count
AP, A/P	anteroposterior
A&P	auscultation and percussion
APAP	acetyl-*para*-aminophenol
APC	acetylsalicylic acid/aspirin, phenacetin, caffeine
aq.	water (*aqua*); aqueous
ARDS	acute respiratory distress syndrome
AROM	active range of motion
AS	aortic stenosis
A.S.	left ear (*auris sinistra*); better to specify "left ear," rather than abbreviating
ASA	acetylsalicylic acid (aspirin)
ASCUS	atypical squamous cells of undetermined significance (abnormal Pap smear finding that does not fully meet the criteria for a cancerous lesion)
ASD	atrial septal defect
ASHD	arteriosclerotic heart disease
AST	aspartate aminotransferase (elevated in liver and heart disease); formerly called serum glutamic-oxaloacetic transaminase (SGOT)

Abbreviations (Continued)

A.U.	both ears (*auris uterque*); better to specify "in each ear/for both ears," rather than abbreviating
Au	gold (*aurum*)
AUB	abnormal uterine bleeding
AV	arteriovenous; atrioventricular
AVM	arteriovenous malformation
AVR	aortic valve replacement
A&W	alive and well
AZT	azidothymidine
B cells	lymphocytes produced in the bone marrow
Ba	barium
BAL	bronchoalveolar lavage
bands	immature white blood cells (granulocytes)
baso	basophils
BBB	bundle branch block
BC	bone conduction
BE	barium enema
bid, b.i.d.	twice a day (*bis in die*)
BKA	below-knee amputation
BM	bowel movement
BMD	bone mineral density
BMR	basal metabolic rate
BMT	bone marrow transplantation
BP, B/P	blood pressure
BPH	benign prostatic hyperplasia/hypertrophy
BPPV	benign paroxysmal positional vertigo
BRBPR	bright red blood per rectum (hematochezia)
BRCA1, BRCA2	breast cancer 1, breast cancer 2 (genetic markers for disease risk)
bs	blood sugar; breath sound(s)
BSE	breast self-examination
BSO	bilateral salpingo-oophorectomy

Abbreviations (Continued)

BSP	Bromsulphalein (bromosulfophthalein)—dye used in liver function testing; its retention is indicative of liver damage or disease
BT	bleeding time
BUN	blood urea nitrogen
bw, BW	birth weight
Bx, bx	biopsy
C	carbon; calorie
°C	degrees Celsius (on "metric" temperature scale); degrees centigrade
c̄	with (*cum*)
C1, C2	first cervical vertebra, second cervical vertebra (and so on)
CA	cancer; carcinoma; cardiac arrest; chronologic age
Ca	calcium
CABG	coronary artery bypass graft/ grafting (cardiovascular surgery)
CAD	coronary artery disease
CAO	chronic airway obstruction
cap	capsule
CAPD	continuous ambulatory peritoneal dialysis
Cath	catheter; catheterization
CBC	complete blood (cell) count
CBT	cognitive behavioral therapy
CC	chief complaint; comorbidity/ complications
cc	cubic centimeter (same as mL: 1/1000 of a liter)
Ccr	creatinine clearance
CCU	coronary care unit; critical care unit
CDC	Centers for Disease Control and Prevention
CDE	complete diagnostic evaluation

Abbreviations (Continued)

CDH	congenital dislocated hip
CEA	carcinoembryonic antigen
cf.	compare (*confer*)
CF	cystic fibrosis; complement fixation (test)
c.gl	with (*cum*) glasses
CGMS	continuous glucose monitoring system
cGy	centigray (1/100 of a gray; a rad)
CHD	coronary heart disease; chronic heart disease
chemo	chemotherapy
CHF	congestive heart failure
chol	cholesterol
chr	chronic
μCi	microcurie
CIN	cervical intraepithelial neoplasia
CIS	carcinoma in situ
CK	creatine kinase
CKD	chronic kidney disease
Cl	chlorine
CLD	chronic liver disease
CLL	chronic lymphocytic leukemia
cm	centimeter (1/100 of a meter)
CMA	certified medical assistant
CMC	carpometacarpal (joint)
CMG	cystometrogram
CML	chronic myelogenous leukemia
CMV	cytomegalovirus
CNS	central nervous system
CO	carbon monoxide; cardiac output
CO_2	carbon dioxide
Co	cobalt
c/o	complains of
COD	condition on discharge
COPD	chronic obstructive pulmonary disease
CP	cerebral palsy; chest pain
CPA	costophrenic angle

Abbreviations (Continued)

CPAP	continuous positive airway pressure
CPD	cephalopelvic disproportion
CPR	cardiopulmonary resuscitation
CR	complete response; cardiorespiratory
CRBSI	catheter-related bloodstream infection
CRF	chronic renal failure
C&S	culture and sensitivity (of sputum)
C-section	cesarean section
CSF	cerebrospinal fluid; colony-stimulating factor
C-spine	cervical spine (films)
CT scan	computed tomography (x-ray imaging in axial and other planes)
ct.	count
CTPA	CT pulmonary angiography
CTS	carpal tunnel syndrome
Cu	copper (*cuprum*)
CVA	cerebrovascular accident; costovertebral angle
CVP	central venous pressure
CVS	cardiovascular system; chorionic villus sampling
c/w	compare with; consistent with
CX, CXR	chest x-ray (film)
Cx	cervix
cysto	cystoscopy
D/C	discontinue
D&C	dilatation/dilation and curettage
DCIS	ductal carcinoma in situ
DD	discharge diagnosis; differential diagnosis
Decub.	decubitus (lying down)
Derm.	dermatology
DES	diethylstilbestrol; diffuse esophageal spasm

Abbreviations (Continued)

DEXA *or* **DXA**	dual-energy x-ray absorptiometry (a test of bone mineral density)
DI	diabetes insipidus; diagnostic imaging
DIC	disseminated intravascular coagulation
DICOM	digital image communication in medicine
diff.	differential count (of kinds of white blood cells)
DIG	digoxin; digitalis
DKA	diabetic ketoacidosis
dL, dl	deciliter (1/10 of a liter)
DLco	diffusion capacity of the lung for carbon monoxide
DLE	discoid lupus erythematosus
DM	diabetes mellitus
DNA	deoxyribonucleic acid
DNR	do not resuscitate
D.O.	doctor of osteopathy
DOA	dead on arrival
DOB	date of birth
DOE	dyspnea on exertion
DPT	diphtheria-pertussis-tetanus (vaccine)
DRE	digital rectal examination
DRG	diagnosis-related group
DSA	digital subtraction angiography
DSM	*Diagnostic and Statistical Manual of Mental Disorders*
DT	delirium tremens (caused by alcohol withdrawal)
DTR	deep tendon reflex(es)
DUB	dysfunctional uterine bleeding
DVT	deep venous thrombosis
D/W	dextrose in water
Dx	diagnosis
EBV	Epstein-Barr virus (cause of mononucleosis)

Abbreviations (Continued)

ECC	endocervical curettage; extracorporeal circulation; emergency cardiac care
ECF	extended care facility
ECG	electrocardiogram
ECHO	echocardiography
ECMO	extracorporeal membrane oxygenation
ECT	electroconvulsive therapy
ED	erectile dysfunction; emergency department
EDC	estimated date of confinement
EEG	electroencephalogram
EENT	eyes, ears, nose, throat
EGD	esophagogastroduodenoscopy
EKG	electrocardiogram
ELISA	enzyme-linked immunosorbent assay
EM	electron microscope
EMB	endometrial biopsy
EMG	electromyogram
EMLA	eutectic mixture of local anesthetics
EMT	emergency medical technician
ENT	ear, nose, throat
EOM	extraocular movement; extraocular muscles
eos	eosinophils (type of white blood cell)
EPO	erythropoietin
ER	emergency room; estrogen receptor
ERCP	endoscopic retrograde cholangiopancreatography
ERT	estrogen replacement therapy
ESR (sed rate)	erythrocyte sedimentation rate (increase indicates inflammation)

Abbreviations (Continued)

ESRD	end-stage renal disease
ESWL	extracorporeal shock wave lithotripsy
ETOH	ethyl alcohol
ETT	exercise tolerance test
EUS	endoscopic ultrasonography
F, °F	Fahrenheit, degrees Fahrenheit
FB	fingerbreadth; foreign body
FBS	fasting blood sugar
FDA	U.S. Food and Drug Administration
FDG-PET	2-deoxy-2[F-18]fluoro-D-glucose positron emission tomography
Fe	iron (*ferrum*)
FEF	forced expiratory flow
FEV$_1$	forced expiratory volume in first second
FH	family history
FHR	fetal heart rate
FPG	fasting plasma glucose
FROM	full range of movement/motion
FSH	follicle-stimulating hormone
F/U	follow-up
5-FU	5-fluorouracil (a chemotherapy drug)
FUO	fever of undetermined origin
Fx	fracture
G	gravida (pregnant)
g, gm	gram
μg	microgram (one millionth of a gram)
g/dL	grams per deciliter
Ga	gallium
GABA	gamma-aminobutyric acid; *also spelled* γ-aminobutyric acid (a neurotransmitter)
GB	gallbladder
GBS	gallbladder series (an x-ray study)
GC	gonococcus

Abbreviations (Continued)

G-CSF	granulocyte colony-stimulating factor (promotes neutrophil production)
Gd	gadolinium
GERD	gastroesophageal reflux disease
GFR	glomerular filtration rate
GH	growth hormone
GI	gastrointestinal
GIST	gastrointestinal stromal tumor
G6PD	glucose-6-phosphate dehydrogenase (enzyme missing in an inherited red blood cell disorder)
GP	general practitioner
GM-CSF	granulocyte-macrophage colony-stimulating factor (promotes myeloid progenitor cells with differentiation to granulocytes)
grav. 1, 2, 3	*gravida* 1, 2, 3—first, second, third pregnancy
gt, gtt	drop (*gutta*), drops (*guttae*)
GTT	glucose tolerance test
GU	genitourinary
Gy	gray—unit of radiation absorption (exposure); equal to 100 rad
GYN, gyn	gynecology
H	hydrogen
h., hr	hour
H$_2$ blocker	histamine H$_2$ receptor antagonist (inhibitor of gastric acid secretion)
HAART	highly active antiretroviral therapy (for AIDS)
HAI	hemagglutination inhibition
Hb, hgb	hemoglobin
HbA$_{1c}$	glycosylated hemoglobin test (for diabetes)
HBV	hepatitis B virus
hCG, HCG	human chorionic gonadotropin

Abbreviations (Continued)

HCl	hydrochloric acid
HCO_3	bicarbonate
Hct, HCT	hematocrit
HCV	hepatitis C virus
HCVD	hypertensive cardiovascular disease
HD	hemodialysis (performed by artificial kidney machine)
HDL	high-density lipoprotein
He	helium
HEENT	head, eyes, ears, nose, throat
Hg	mercury
H&H	hematocrit and hemoglobin (measurement)—red blood cell tests
HIPAA	Health Insurance Portability and Accountability Act (of 1996)
HIV	human immunodeficiency virus
HLA	histocompatibility locus antigen (identifies cells as "self")
HNP	herniated nucleus pulposus
h/o	history of
H_2O	water
H&P	history and physical (examination)
HPF; hpf	high-power field (in microscopy)
HPI	history of present illness
HPV	human papillomavirus
HRT	hormone replacement therapy
hs	half-strength
h.s.	at bedtime (*hora somni*)—write out so as not to confuse with hs (half-strength)
HSG	hysterosalpingography
HSV	herpes simplex virus
ht	height
HTN	hypertension (high blood pressure)
Hx	history
I	iodine
^{131}I	a radioactive isotope of iodine

Abbreviations (Continued)

IBD	inflammatory bowel disease (Crohn's and ulcerative colitis)
ICD	implantable cardioverter-defibrillator
ICP	intracranial pressure
ICSH	interstitial cell–stimulating hormone
ICU	intensive care unit
ID	infectious disease
I&D	incision and drainage
IgA, IgD, IgE, IgG, IgM	immunoglobulins (type of antibodies)
IHD	ischemic heart disease
IHSS	idiopathic hypertrophic subaortic stenosis
IL-1 to IL-15	interleukins
IM	intramuscular; infectious mononucleosis
inf.	infusion; inferior
INH	isoniazid (a drug used to treat tuberculosis)
inj.	injection
I&O	intake and output (measurement of patient's fluids)
IOL	intraocular lens (implant)
IOP	intraocular pressure
IPPB	intermittent positive-pressure breathing
IQ	intelligence quotient
ITP	idiopathic thrombocytopenic purpura
IUD	intrauterine device
IUP	intrauterine pregnancy
IV	intravenous
IVP	intravenous pyelogram
K	potassium
kg	kilogram (equal to 1000 g)

Abbreviations (Continued)

KJ	knee jerk
KS	Kaposi sarcoma
KUB	kidneys, ureters, bladder (x-ray study)
L, l	liter; left; lower
µL	microliter (one millionth of a liter)
L1, L2	first lumbar vertebra, second lumbar vertebra (and so on)
LA	left atrium
LAD	left anterior descending (coronary artery); lymphadenopathy
LADA	latent autoimmune diabetes in adults
lat	lateral
LB	large bowel
LBBB	left bundle branch block (a form of heart block)
LBW	low birth weight
LD	lethal dose
LDH	lactate dehydrogenase
LDL	low-density lipoprotein (high levels are associated with heart disease)
L-dopa	levodopa (a drug used to treat Parkinson disease)
LE	lupus erythematosus
LEEP	loop electrocautery excision procedure
LES	lower esophageal sphincter
LFTs	liver function tests
LH	luteinizing hormone
LLL	left lower lobe (of lung)
LLQ	left lower quadrant (of abdomen)
LMP	last menstrual period
LMWH	low-molecular-weight heparin
LOC	loss of consciousness
LOS	length of (hospital) stay
LP	lumbar puncture
lpf	low-power field (in microscopy)

Abbreviations (Continued)

LPN	licensed practical nurse
LS	lumbosacral spine
LSD	lysergic acid diethylamide (a hallucinogen)
LSH	laparoscopic supracervical hysterectomy
LSK	liver, spleen, kidneys
LTB	laryngotracheal bronchitis (croup)
LTC	long-term care
LTH	luteotropic hormone (same as prolactin)
LUL	left upper lobe (of lung)
LUQ	left upper quadrant (of abdomen)
LV	left ventricle
LVAD	left ventricular assist device
L&W	living and well
lymphs	lymphocytes
lytes	electrolytes
MA	mental age
MAC	monitored anesthesia care; *Mycobacterium avium* complex (a common cause of opportunistic pneumonia)
MAI	*Mycobacterium avium-intracellulare*
MAOI	monoamine oxidase inhibitor (a type of antidepressant)
MBD	minimal brain dysfunction
mcg	microgram—also abbreviated µg; equal to one millionth of a gram
MCH	mean corpuscular hemoglobin (average amount in each red blood cell)
MCHC	mean corpuscular hemoglobin concentration (average concentration in a single red cell)
mCi	millicurie
µCi	microcurie

Abbreviations (Continued)

MCP	metacarpophalangeal (joint)
MCV	mean corpuscular volume (average size of a single red blood cell)
M.D.	doctor of medicine
MDI	multiple daily injections; metered-dose inhaler (used to deliver aerosolized medication to a patient)
MDR	minimum daily requirement
MDS	myelodysplastic syndrome (a bone marrow disorder)
MED	minimum effective dose
mEq	milliequivalent
mEq/L	milliequivalent per liter (unit of measure for the concentration of a solution)
mets	metastases
MG	myasthenia gravis
Mg	magnesium
mg	milligram (1/1000 of a gram)
mg/cc^3	milligram per cubic centimeter
mg/dL	milligram per deciliter
MH	marital history; mental health
MI	myocardial infarction; mitral insufficiency
mL, ml	milliliter (1/1000 of a liter)
mm	millimeter (1/1000 of a meter; 0.039 inch)
mm Hg, mmHg	millimeters of mercury
MMPI	Minnesota Multiphasic Personality Inventory
MMR	measles-mumps-rubella (vaccine)
MMT	manual muscle testing
μm	micrometer (one millionth of a meter, or 1/1000 of a millimeter); sometimes seen in older sources as μ (for "micron," an outdated term)
MoAb	monoclonal antibody

Abbreviations (Continued)

MODS	multiple organ dysfunction syndrome
monos	monocytes (type of white blood cells)
MR	mitral regurgitation; magnetic resonance
MRA	magnetic resonance angiography
MRI	magnetic resonance imaging
mRNA	messenger RNA
MRSA	methicillin-resistant *Staphylococcus aureus*
MS	multiple sclerosis; mitral stenosis; morphine sulfate
MSL	midsternal line
MTD	maximum tolerated dose
MTX	methotrexate
MUGA	multiple-gated acquisition scan (of heart)
multip	multipara; multiparous
MVP	mitral valve prolapse
myop	myopia (nearsightedness)
N	nitrogen
NA, N/A	not applicable; not available
Na	sodium (*natrium*)
NB	newborn
NBS	normal bowel sounds; normal breath sounds
ND	normal delivery; normal development
NED	no evidence of disease
neg.	negative
NG tube	nasogastric tube
NHL	non-Hodgkin lymphoma
NICU	neonatal intensive care unit
NK cells	natural killer cells
NKA	no known allergies
NKDA	no known drug allergies
NOTES	natural orifice transluminal endoscopic surgery

Abbreviations (Continued)

NPO	nothing by mouth (*nil per os*)
NSAID	nonsteroidal anti-inflammatory drug (often prescribed to treat musculoskeletal disorders)
NSR	normal sinus rhythm (of heart)
NTP	normal temperature and pressure
O, O₂	oxygen
OA	osteoarthritis
OB/GYN	obstetrics and gynecology
OCPs	oral contraceptive pills
O.D.	doctor of optometry; right eye (*oculus dexter*); better to specify "right eye," rather than abbreviating
OD	overdose
OMT	osteopathic manipulative treatment
OR	operating room
ORIF	open reduction plus internal fixation
ORTH; Ortho.	orthopedics
OS	left eye (*oculus sinister*); better to specify "left eye," rather than abbreviating
os	opening; bone
OT	occupational therapy (helps patients perform activities of daily living and function in work-related situations)
OU	both eyes (*oculus uterque*); better to specify "both eyes," rather than abbreviating
oz	ounce
P	phosphorus; posterior; pressure; pulse; pupil
p̄	after
P2, P₂	pulmonary valve closure (a heart sound)
PA	pulmonary artery; posteroanterior

Abbreviations (Continued)

P-A	posteroanterior
P&A	percussion and auscultation
PAC	premature atrial contraction
Paco$_2$	partial pressure of carbon dioxide in arterial blood
PACS	picture archival communications system
PAD	peripheral arterial disease
palp.	palpable; palpation
PALS	pediatric advanced life support
Pao$_2$	partial pressure of oxygen in blood
Pap smear	Papanicolaou smear (from cervix and vagina)
para 1, 2, 3	unipara, bipara, tripara (number of viable births)
pc, p.c.	after meals (*post cibum*)
PCA	patient-controlled anesthesia
PCI	percutaneous coronary intervention
Pco$_2$, pCO$_2$	partial pressure of carbon dioxide
PCP	*Pneumocystis* pneumonia; phencyclidine (a hallucinogen)
PCR	polymerase chain reaction (process that allows making copies of genes)
PD	peritoneal dialysis
PDA	patent ductus arteriosus
PDR	*Physicians' Desk Reference*
PE	physical examination; pulmonary embolus
PEEP	positive end-expiratory pressure
PEG	percutaneous endoscopic gastrostomy (feeding tube placed in stomach)
PEJ	percutaneous endoscopic jejunostomy (feeding tube placed in small intestine)
per os	by mouth

Abbreviations (Continued)

PERRLA	pupils equal, round, reactive to light and accommodation
PET	positron emission tomography
PE tube	ventilating tube for eardrum
PFT	pulmonary function test
PG	prostaglandin
PH	past history
pH	potential hydrogen (scale to indicate degree of acidity or alkalinity)
PI	present illness
PICC	peripherally inserted central catheter
PID	pelvic inflammatory disease
PIN	prostatic intraepithelial neoplasia
PIP	proximal interphalangeal (joint)
PKU	phenylketonuria
PM, p.m., PM	in the afternoon (*post meridiem*)
PMH	past medical history
PMN	polymorphonuclear leukocyte
PMS	premenstrual syndrome
PND	paroxysmal nocturnal dyspnea
PNS	peripheral nervous system
PO, p.o.	by mouth (*per os*)
p/o	postoperative
Po$_2$, po$_2$	partial pressure of oxygen
poly	polymorphonuclear leukocyte
postop	postoperative (after surgery)
PPBS	postprandial blood sugar
PPD	purified protein derivative (used in test for tuberculosis)
preop	preoperative
prep	prepare for
PR	partial response
primip	primipara
PRL	prolactin
p.r.n.	as needed; as necessary (*pro re nata*)
procto	proctoscopy
prot.	protocol

Abbreviations (Continued)

Pro. time	prothrombin time (test of blood clotting)
PSA	prostate-specific antigen
PT	prothrombin time; physical therapy (helps patients regain use of muscles and joints after injury or surgery)
pt.	patient
PTA	prior to admission (to hospital)
PTC	percutaneous transhepatic cholangiography
PTCA	percutaneous transluminal coronary angioplasty
PTH	parathyroid hormone
PTHC	percutaneous transhepatic cholangiography
PTSD	post-traumatic stress disorder
PTT	partial thromboplastin time (a test of blood clotting)
PU	pregnancy urine
PUVA	psoralen ultraviolet A (a treatment for psoriasis)
PVC	premature ventricular contraction
PVD	peripheral vascular disease
PVT	paroxysmal ventricular tachycardia
PWB	partial weight-bearing
Px	prognosis
Q	blood volume; rate of blood flow (daily)
q	every (*quaque*, "each")
qAM	every morning; better to specify than to abbreviate
qd, q.d.	every day (*quaque die*); better to specify "each/every day," rather than confusing with qid or qod
qh	every hour (*quaque hora*); better to specify than to abbreviate

Abbreviations (Continued)

q2h	every 2 hours; better to specify than to abbreviate
qid	four times daily (*quater in die*); better to specify than to abbreviate
q.n.s.	quantity not sufficient (*quantum non sufficit*)
qod	every other day; better to specify than to abbreviate
qPM	every evening; better to specify than to abbreviate
QRS	a wave complex in an electrocardiographic study
q.s.	sufficient quantity (*quantum sufficit*)
qt	quart
R	respiration; right
RA	rheumatoid arthritis; right atrium
Ra	radium
rad	radiation absorbed dose
RAIU	radioactive iodine uptake test
RBBB	right bundle branch block
RBC, rbc	red blood count; red blood cell
RDDA	recommended daily dietary allowance
RDS	respiratory distress syndrome
REM	rapid eye movement
RF	rheumatoid factor
Rh (factor)	rhesus (monkey) factor in blood
RhoGAM	drug to prevent Rh factor reaction in Rh-negative women
RIA	radioimmunoassay (test for measuring minute quantities of a substance)
RLL	right lower lobe/lung
RLQ	right lower quadrant (abdomen)
RML	right middle lobe (lung)
RNA	ribonucleic acid
R/O	rule out

Abbreviations (Continued)

ROM	range of motion
ROS	review of systems
RRR	regular rate and rhythm (of heart)
RT	right; radiation therapy
RUL	right upper lobe (of lung)
RUQ	right upper quadrant (of abdomen)
RV	right ventricle
R̄x	treatment; therapy; prescription
s̄	without (*sine*)
S1, S2	first sacral vertebra, second sacral vertebra (and so on)
S-A node	sinoatrial node (pacemaker of heart)
SAD	seasonal affective disorder
SARS	severe acute respiratory syndrome
SBE	subacute bacterial endocarditis
SBFT	small bowel follow-through (x-ray study of small intestine function)
segs	segmented, mature white blood cells (neutrophils)
SERM	selective estrogen receptor modulator
s.gl	without (*sine*) glasses
SGOT	*see* AST
SGPT	*see* ALT
SIADH	syndrome of inappropriate antidiuretic hormone
SIDS	sudden infant death syndrome
Sig.	directions—medication instructions (*signa,* "mark")
SIRS	systemic inflammatory response syndrome (severe bacteremia)
SL	sublingual
SLE	systemic lupus erythematosus
SMA-12	blood chemistry profile including 12 different studies/assays

Abbreviations (Continued)

SMAC	sequential multiple analyzer computer (automated analytical device for testing blood)
SOAP	subjective, objective, assessment, plan (used for patient notes)
SOB	shortness of breath
s.o.s.	if necessary (*si opus sit*, "if there should be [such a] necessity")
S/P	status post (previous disease, condition, or procedure)
sp. gr.	specific gravity
SPECT	single photon emission computed tomography
SQ	subcutaneous
S/S, Sx	signs and symptoms
SSCP	substernal chest pain
SSRI	selective serotonin reuptake inhibitor (a type of antidepressant)
Staph.	staphylococci (berry-shaped bacteria in clusters
stat., STAT	immediately (*statim*)
STD	sexually transmitted disease
STH	somatotropic hormone (somatotropin) (a growth hormone
STI	sexually transmitted infection
Strep.	streptococci (berry-shaped bacteria in twisted chains)
sub-Q	subcutaneously
SVC	superior vena cava
SVD	spontaneous vaginal delivery
Sx	symptoms; signs and symptoms
Sz	seizure
T	temperature; time
T cells	lymphocytes produced in the thymus gland
T tube	tube placed in biliary tract for drainage

Abbreviations (Continued)

T1, T2	first thoracic vertebra, second thoracic vertebra (and so on)
T$_3$	triiodothyronine (test)
T$_4$	thyroxine (test)
TA	therapeutic abortion
T&A	tonsillectomy and adenoidectomy
TAB	therapeutic abortion
TAH	total abdominal hysterectomy
TAT	Thematic Apperception Test
TB	tuberculosis
Tc	technetium
TEE	transesophageal echocardiogram
TENS	transcutaneous electrical nerve stimulation
TFT	thyroid function test
THR	total hip replacement (an arthroplasty procedure)
TIA	transient ischemic attack
tid, t.i.d.	three times daily (*ter in die*)
TKR	total knee replacement (an arthroplasty procedure)
TLC	total lung capacity
TLE	temporal lobe epilepsy
TM	tympanic membrane
TMJ	temporomandibular joint
TNF	tumor necrosis factor
TNM	tumor-node-metastasis (cancer staging system)
tPA	tissue plasminogen activator
TPN	total parenteral nutrition
TPR	temperature, pulse, respirations
TRUS	transrectal ultrasound (examination) (test to access the prostate and guide precise placement of a biopsy needle)
TSH	thyroid-stimulating hormone
TSS	toxic shock syndrome
TUR, TURP	transurethral resection of the prostate

Abbreviations (Continued)

TVH	total vaginal hysterectomy
Tx	treatment
UA	urinalysis; unstable angina (chest pain at rest or of increasing frequency)
UAO	upper airway obstruction
UC	uterine contraction(s)
UE	upper extremity
UGI	upper gastrointestinal
umb.	navel (*umbilicus*)
U/O	urinary output
URI	upper respiratory infection
U/S	ultrasound; ultrasonography
UTI	urinary tract infection
UV	ultraviolet
VA	visual acuity
VATS	video-assisted thoracic surgery
VC	vital capacity (of lungs)
VCUG	voiding cystourethrogram
VDRL	Venereal Disease Research Laboratory (test for syphilis)
VEGF	vascular endothelial growth factor
VF	visual field; ventricular fibrillation
V/Q scan	ventilation-perfusion scan (of lung)
V/S	vital signs; versus
VSD	ventricular septal defect
VT	ventricular tachycardia (an abnormal heart rhythm)
VTE	venous thromboembolism
WAIS	Wechsler Adult Intelligence Scale
WBC, wbc	white blood cell; white blood count
WDWN	well developed and well nourished
WISC	Wechsler Intelligence Scale for Children
WNL	within normal limits
wt	weight
XRT	radiation therapy
y/o, yr	year(s) old

Acronyms*

An *acronym* is the name for an abbreviation that forms a pronounceable word.

ACE (ace)	angiotensin-converting enzyme
AIDS (aydz)	acquired immunodeficiency syndrome
APGAR (ap-gahr)	appearance, pulse, grimace, activity, respiration
BUN (bun *or* bee-yu-en)	blood urea nitrogen
CABG (cabbage)	coronary artery bypass graft/grafting
CAT (cat)	computerized axial tomography (*outdated term; use* CT)
CPAP (see-pap)	continuous positive airway pressure
DEXA (decksa)	dual energy X-ray absorptiometry
ELISA (eliza)	enzyme-linked immunosorbent assay
GERD (gerd)	gastroesophageal reflux disease
GIST (jist)	gastrointestinal stromal tumor
HAART (heart)	highly active antiretroviral therapy
HIPAA (hip-ah)	Health Insurance Portability and Accountability Act of 1996
LASER (lay-zer)	light amplification by stimulated emission of radiation
LASIK (lay-sik)	laser in *situ* keratomileusis

---

*From Chabner DE: The Language of Medicine, 9th ed. Philadelphia, Saunders, 2011.

LEEP (leap)	loop electrocautery excision procedure
MAC (mak)	monitored anesthesia care; *mycobacterium avium* complex
MICU (mik-yu)	medical intensive care unit
MIS (miss)	minimally invasive surgery
MODS (modz)	multiple organ dysfunction syndrome
MUGA (mugah)	multiple-gated acquisition (scan)
NSAID (n-sed)	nonsteroidal anti-inflammatory drug
NICU (nik-u)	neonatal intensive care unit
PACS (paks)	picture archival communications system
PALS (palz)	pediatric advanced life support
PEEP (peep)	positive end-expiratory pressure
PEG (peg)	percutaneous endoscopic gastrostomy
PERRLA (per-lah)	pupils equal, round, reactive to light and accommodation
PET (pet)	positron emission tomography
PICU (pik-yu)	pediatric intensive care unit
PIP (pip)	proximal interphalangeal (joint)
PUVA (poo-vah)	psoralen ultraviolet A
REM (rem)	rapid eye movement
SAD (sad)	seasonal affective disorder
SARS (sahrz)	severe acute respiratory syndrome
SERM (serm)	selective estrogen receptor modulator
SICU (sik-u)	surgical intensive care unit
SIDS (sidz)	sudden infant death syndrome

SIRS (serz)	systemic inflammatory response syndrome
SMAC (smack)	sequential multiple analyzer computer (blood testing)
SOAP (soap)	subjective, objective, assessment, plan
SPECT (spekt)	single photon emission computed tomography
TENS (tenz)	transcutaneous electrical nerve stimulation
TRUS (truss)	transrectal ultrasound
TURP (turp)	transurethral resection of the prostate
VATS (vatz)	video-assisted thoracic surgery

Eponyms*

Achilles tendon (Achilles, Greek mythological hero)	This tendon connects the calf muscles to the heel. It lies at the only part of Achilles' body that was still vulnerable after his mother dipped him as an infant into the river Styx, when she held him by the heel.
Alzheimer disease (Alois Alzheimer, MD, German neurologist, 1864–1915)	Progressive mental deterioration marked by confusion, memory failure, and disorientation.
Apgar score (Virginia Apgar, MD, American anesthesiologist, 1909–1974)	Evaluation of an infant's physical condition, usually performed 1 minute and then 5 minutes after birth. Highest score is 10. An Apgar rating of 9/10 is a score of 9 at 1 minute and 10 at 5 minutes.

---

*From Chabner DE: The Language of Medicine, 9th ed. Philadelphia, Saunders, 2011.

Asperger syndrome (Hans Asperger, Austrian psychiatrist, 1906–1980)	Developmental disorder characterized by impairment of social interactions (resembling autism) but lacking delays in language development and mental functioning.
Barrett esophagus (Norman Barrett, MD, Australian thoracic surgeon, 1903–1979)	Abnormal growth of cells at the distal end of the esophagus, often as a result of damage from gastroesophageal reflux disease (GERD).
Bell palsy (Charles Bell, Scottish surgeon, 1774–1842)	Unilateral (one-sided) paralysis of the facial nerve.
Burkitt lymphoma (Denis Burkitt, English surgeon in Africa, 1911–1993)	Malignant tumor of lymph nodes; chiefly seen in central Africa. The Epstein-Barr virus is associated with this lymphoma.
Cheyne-Stokes respiration (John Cheyne, Scottish physician, 1777–1836, and William Stokes, Irish physician 1804–1878)	Abnormal pattern of breathing with alternating periods of stoppage of breathing and deep, rapid breathing.
Colles fracture (Abraham Colles, Irish surgeon, 1773–1843)	Break (fracture) of the radius (outer forearm bone) near the wrist.

Crohn disease (Burrill B. Crohn, American physician, 1884–1983)	Chronic inflammatory bowel disease of unknown origin; usually affecting the ileum (last part of the small intestine), colon, or any part of the gastrointestinal tract.
Cushing syndrome (Harvey W. Cushing, American surgeon, 1869–1939)	Disorder resulting from chronic, excessive production of cortisol from the adrenal cortex. It can also result from administration of glucocorticoids (cortisone) in large doses for long periods of time.
Duchenne muscular dystrophy (Guillaume Benjamin Amand Duchenne, French neurologist, 1806–1875)	Abnormal, inherited condition marked by progressive hardening of muscles in the leg and hips (pelvis) beginning in infancy.
Epstein-Barr virus (Michael A. Epstein, English pathologist, born 1921; Yvonne M. Barr, English virologist, born 1932)	The herpesvirus that causes infectious mononucleosis and is associated with malignant conditions such as nose and throat cancer, Burkitt's lymphoma, and Hodgkin's disease.
eustachian tube (Bartolomeo Eustachio, Italian anatomist, 1524–1574)	Anatomic passageway that joins the throat and the middle ear cavity.

Ewing sarcoma (James Ewing, American pathologist, 1866–1943)	Malignant tumor that develops from bone marrow, usually in long bones or the hip (pelvis).
fallopian tube (Gabriele Falloppio, Italian anatomist, 1523–1562)	One of a pair of tubes or ducts leading from the ovary to the upper portion of the uterus.
Foley catheter (Frederic Foley, American physician, 1891–1966)	Rubber tube that is placed in the urethra to provide drainage of urine.
Giardia (Alfred Giardia, French biologist, 1846–1908)	One-celled organism (protozoon) that causes gastrointestinal infection with diarrhea, abdominal cramps, and weight loss. Cause of infection is usually fecally contaminated water.
Hodgkin disease (Thomas Hodgkin, English physician, 1798–1866)	Malignant tumor of the lymph nodes.
Huntington disease (George S. Huntington, American physician, 1851–1916)	Rare, hereditary condition marked by chronic, progressively worsening dance-like movements (chorea) and mental deterioration, resulting in dementia.

Kaposi sarcoma (Moricz Kaposi, Austrian dermatologist, 1837–1902)	Malignant neoplasm of cells that line blood and lymph vessels. Soft brownish or purple papules appear on the skin. The tumor can metastasize to lymph nodes and internal organs. It is often associated with AIDS.
Marfan syndrome (Bernard-Jean A. Marfan, French pediatrician, 1858–1942)	Hereditary condition that affects bones, muscles, the cardiovascular system (leading to aneurysms), and eyes (lens dislocation). Affected people have overlong extremities with "spider-like" fingers (arachnodactyly), underdeveloped muscles, and easily movable joints.
Ménière disease (Prosper Ménière, French physician, 1799–1862)	Chronic disease of the inner ear with recurrent episodes of dizziness (vertigo), hearing loss, and ringing in the ears (tinnitus).
Neisseria gonorrhoeae (Albert L. S. Neisser, Polish dermatologist, 1855–1916)	Type of bacterium that causes gonorrhea (sexually transmitted disease).

Paget disease (James Paget, English surgeon, 1814–1899)	Disease of bone, often affecting middle-aged or elderly people; marked by bone destruction and poor bone repair.
Pap test (George Papanicolaou, Greek physician in the United States, 1883–1962)	Method of examining stained cells obtained from the cervix and vagina. It is a common way to detect cervical cancer.
Parkinson disease (James Parkinson, English physician, 1755–1824)	Slowly progressive degenerative neurologic disorder marked by tremors, mask-like facial appearance, shuffling gait (manner of walking), and muscle rigidity and weakness.
Raynaud phenomenon (Maurice Raynaud, French physician, 1834–1881)	Intermittent attacks of loss of blood flow (ischemia) of the extremities of the body (fingers, toes, ears, and nose). Episodes most often are caused by exposure to cold.
Reye syndrome (R. Douglas Reye, Austrian pathologist, 1912–1978)	Acute brain disease (encephalopathy) and disease of internal organs after an acute viral infection.
Rinne test (Heinrich A. Rinne, German otologist, 1819–1868)	Hearing test using a vibrating tuning fork placed against a bone behind the patient's ear (mastoid bone).

Rorschach test (Herman Rorschach, Swiss psychiatrist, 1884–1922)	Personality test based on the patient's interpretation of 10 standard ink blots.
Salmonella (Daniel E. Salmon, American pathologist, 1850–1914)	Type of bacteria (rod-shaped) that causes typhoid fever and types of gastroenteritis (inflammation of the stomach and intestines).
Shigella (Kiyoshi Shiga, Japanese bacteriologist, 1870–1957)	Type of bacteria that causes severe infectious gastroenteritis (inflammation of stomach and intestines) and dysentery (diarrhea, abdominal pain, and fever).
Sjögren syndrome (Heinrik S. C. Sjögren, Swedish ophthalmologist, 1899–1986)	Abnormal dryness of the mouth, eyes, and mucous membranes, caused by deficient fluid production. It is a disorder of the immune system.
Snellen test (Herman Snellen, Dutch ophthalmologist, 1834–1908)	Test of visual clarity (acuity) using a special chart. Letters, numbers, or symbols are arranged on the chart in decreasing size from top to bottom.

Tay-Sachs disease (Warren Tay, English ophthalmologist, 1843–1927, and Bernard Sachs, American neurologist, 1858–1944)	Inherited disorder of nerve degeneration caused by deficiency of an enzyme. Most affected children die between the ages of 2 and 4 years.
Tourette syndrome (Georges Gilles de la Tourette, French neurologist, 1857–1927)	Condition marked by abnormal facial grimaces, inappropriate speech, and involuntary movements of eyes, arms, and shoulders (tics).
von Willebrand disease (Erick A. von Willebrand, Finnish physician, 1870–1949)	Inherited blood disorder marked by abnormally slow blood clotting; caused by deficiency in a blood clotting factor (factor VIII).
Weber tuning fork test (Hermann D. Weber, English physician, 1823–1918)	Test of hearing using a vibrating tuning fork with the stem placed in the center of the patient's forehead.
Whipple procedure (Allen O. Whipple, American surgeon, 1881–1963)	Surgical procedure to remove a portion of the pancreas and the stomach and the entire first part of the small intestine (duodenum). Used in the treatment of pancreatic cancer and other conditions.
Wilms tumor (Max Wilms, German surgeon, 1867–1918)	Malignant tumor of the kidney occurring in young children.

Symbols*

=	equals
≠	does not equal
+	positive
−	negative
↑	above, increase
↓	below, decrease
♀	female
♂	male
→	to (in direction of)
>	(is) greater than; better to write out than to use symbol
<	(is) less than; better to write out than to use symbol
1°	primary to
2°	secondary to
ʒ	dram
ℨ	ounce
%	percent
°	degree; hour
:	ratio; "is to"
±	plus or minus (either positive or negative)
′	foot
″	inch
∴	therefore
@	at, each; better to write out than to use symbol
c̄	with

*From Chabner DE: The Language of Medicine, 9th ed. Philadelphia, Saunders, 2011.

$\bar{s}$	without
#	pound; number
$\cong$	approximately equals, is about
Δ	change
p	short arm of a chromosome
q	long arm of a chromosome

Plurals*

The rules commonly used to form plurals of medical terms are as follows:

1. For words ending in **a**, retain the **a** and add **e**.
   Examples:

SINGULAR	PLURAL
vertebra	vertebrae
bursa	bursae
bulla	bullae

2. For words ending in **is**, drop the **is** and add **es**.
   Examples:

SINGULAR	PLURAL
anastomosis	anastomoses
metastasis	metastases
epiphysis	epiphyses
prosthesis	prostheses
pubis	pubes

3. For words ending in **ex** and **ix**, drop the **ex** or **ix** and add **ices**.
   Examples:

SINGULAR	PLURAL
apex	apices
varix	varices

4. For words ending in **on**, drop the **on** and add **a**.
   Examples:

SINGULAR	PLURAL
ganglion	ganglia
spermatozoon	spermatozoa

---

*From Chabner DE: The Language of Medicine, 9th ed. Philadelphia, Saunders, 2011.

5. For words ending in **um**, drop the **um** and add **a**.
   Examples:

SINGULAR	PLURAL
bacterium	bacteria
diverticulum	diverticula
ovum	ova

6. For words ending in **us**, drop the **us** and add **i**.
   Examples:

SINGULAR	PLURAL
calculus	calculi
bronchus	bronchi
nucleus	nuclei

   Two exceptions to this rule are vir<u>uses</u> and sin<u>uses</u>.

7. Additional rules are used to form plurals in other word families.
   Examples:

SINGULAR	PLURAL
forame<u>n</u>	foram<u>ina</u>
iri<u>s</u>	ir<u>ides</u>
fem<u>ur</u>	fem<u>ora</u>
anomal<u>y</u>	anoma<u>lies</u>
biops<u>y</u>	biops<u>ies</u>
aden<u>oma</u>	adeno<u>mata</u>

Medical Terms Easily Confused

Health care professionals who have difficulty with the English language may face particular challenges with terms commonly used in the health care setting. The unique application of words with very specific meanings may be a source of confusion.

The words and phrases in the following list have been identified as frequently causing problems because of similarities in pronunciation or spelling. Entries are presented in pairs or in groups of three or four terms, as appropriate, so that the reader may compare and contrast spellings and definitions of similar-sounding or -appearing words and phrases.

TERM	DEFINITION
abduction	moving away from (often dictated as "A-B-DUC-tion")
adduction	moving toward (often dictated as "A-D-DUC-tion")
absorption	taking up or in of a substance
adsorption	attracting and holding substances at the surface
acetic	sour (as vinegar or acetic acid)
acidic	pertaining to an acid; acid-forming
afferent	carrying toward a center
efferent	carrying away from a center
alkalosis	increased alkalinity of blood and tissues
ankylosis	condition of joint stiffening or immobilization

TERM	DEFINITION
ante- anti-	before; in front of against
anuresis enuresis	retention of urine in the bladder ("condition without urine") involuntary discharge of urine; bed-wetting
aphagia aphakia aphasia aplasia	inability to swallow absence of the lens of the eye (as after extraction of a cataract) inability to speak or inability to comprehend spoken or written language lack of development of an organ or tissue
arterio arthr/o ather/o	artery joint plaque (fatty substance)
ascitic asthenic	pertaining to fluid accumulation in the abdomen (ascites) pertaining to a lack or loss of energy
aura aural oral	sensation that precedes a seizure pertaining to the ear pertaining to the mouth
auxiliary axillary	giving assistance or support pertaining to the armpit
bisect resect transect dissect	cut in half cut out (remove) cut across cut apart or separate
blephar/o phleb/o	eyelid vein

TERM	DEFINITION
bolus	single large mass or quantity of drug or medication that is administered orally or intravenously
bullous	pertaining to bullae (large blisters)
caliber	diameter of a canal or tube; diameter of a bullet
calipers	instrument used to measure thickness or diameter of a solid
callous	hard (as the nature of a callus)
callus	the epidermis (skin); network of woven bone formed at the ends of a broken bone
canker sore	ulceration on the mucous membrane of the mouth
chancre	primary lesion of syphilis (SH{short-A}NK-{short-e}r)
carotid	artery of the neck
parotid	salivary gland near the ear
cecal	pertaining to the cecum (first part of the colon)
fecal	pertaining to feces (solid wastes)
thecal	pertaining to a sheath or enclosing case
-centesis	surgical puncture to remove fluid
-cyesis	pregnancy
-genesis	producing or forming

TERM	DEFINITION
cerebellum	posterior portion of the brain (responsible for balance)
cerebrum	largest part of the brain (responsible for thought, memory, sensations, speech, vision, movement)
chol/e	bile; gall
chol/o	colon (large intestine)
cholic	pertaining to bile
colic	pertaining to acute abdominal pain
chrono	time
coron/o	heart
cirrhosal	pertaining to cirrhosis (liver disease)
serosal	pertaining to a serosa (thin membranous covering)
scirrhous	pertaining to hard mass or tumor
serous	pertaining to serum (clear portion of blood minus cells and clotting proteins)
cirrhosis	liver disease
xerosis	condition of dryness
CNS	central nervous system
C&S	culture and sensitivity
coccyx	tailbone
-cocci	berry-shaped bacteria
creatine	high-energy phosphate compound present in muscle
creatinine	nitrogenous waste product excreted in urine
cyst/o	urinary
cyt/o	cell

TERM	DEFINITION
cytotoxin	a poison (toxin) or an antibody with a toxic effect on cells
Cytoxan	drug used in chemotherapy
diverticulitis	inflammation of diverticula
diverticulosis	abnormal condition of presence of diverticula
diarrhea	abnormally frequent and loose bowel movements
diuresis	excretion of abnormally large quantity of urine
-dipsia	thirst
-pepsia	digestion
dysphagia	difficulty in swallowing
dysphasia	difficulty in speaking
dysplasia	abnormal formation (development)
-emia	blood condition
-penia	deficiency
-pnea	breathing
endemic	indigenous to a geographic area or population
epidemic	affecting large numbers of people at the same time
pandemic	affecting the population of a country, a people, or the world
esotropia	inward turning of the eye; cross-eye
exotropia	outward turning of the eye; wall-eye
facial	pertaining to the face
fascial	pertaining to fascia (connective tissue)
faucial	pertaining to the passageway from the mouth to the pharynx

TERM	DEFINITION
fovea	cup-shaped pit or depression (central section of the retina of the eye)
phobia	persistent, irrational, intense fear
glands	groups of cells specialized to function as secretory or excretory structures
glans	a small, rounded structure, as the glans penis (tip of the organ)
graft	tissue implanted from one place to another
graph	instrument to record data
hematoma	collection of blood (bruise)
hepatoma	malignant tumor of the liver
hemodialysis	artificial kidney machine to filter waste from blood
hemolysis	destruction of red blood cells
hemostasis	stopping the flow of blood
homeostasis	maintaining a constant environment
ileac	pertaining to the third part of the small intestine (ileum)
iliac	pertaining to the upper portion of the hip bone (ilium)
ileum	third part of small intestine
ilium	superior portion of hip bone
ileus	obstruction of the intestine
inter-	between
infra-	below, beneath
intra-	within
in vitro	within a test tube ("in glass")
in vivo	within a living organism

TERM	DEFINITION
labial	pertaining to a lip or lip-like structure
labile	unstable; gliding from point to point
lice	parasites (*singular is* louse)
lyse	to cause disintegration of a substance
-malacia	softening
malaise	bodily discomfort
malleolus	bony prominence on either side of the ankle joint
malleus	small bone in the middle portion of the ear
mammoplasty	surgical repair of the breast
manoplasty	plastic surgery of the hand
meiosis	type of cell division to form gametes or sex cells (egg and sperm)
miosis	contraction of the pupil of the eye
mitosis	type of cell division resulting in the formation of identical daughter cells
mycosis	abnormal condition of fungi in the body (mold or yeast infection)
miotic	drug that causes contraction of the pupil of the eye
myopic	pertaining to being nearsighted (myopia)
menorrhagia	excessive uterine bleeding during menstruation
metrorrhagia	abnormal uterine bleeding not during menstruation
menometrorrhagia	excessive uterine bleeding both during menstruation and at other times

TERM	DEFINITION
mucous	pertaining to or resembling mucus
mucus	secretion from mucous membranes
myeloma	malignant tumor of the bone marrow
myoma	benign tumor of muscle
my/o	muscle
myx/o	mucus
odont/o	tooth
orth/o	straight
or/o	mouth
ox/o	oxygen
palmar	pertaining to the palm of the hand
plantar	pertaining to the sole of the foot
palpable	able to be felt with a hand
palpebral	pertaining to the eyelid
palpation	touching, feeling, or examination with hands and fingers
palpitation	rapid pulsation of the heart
-penia	deficiency
-pnea	breathing
per-	through
peri-	surrounding
perineal	pertaining to the perineum (genital area in female and male)
peritoneal	pertaining to the peritoneum (membrane surrounding the abdominal organs)
peroneal	pertaining to the fibula (smaller of two lower leg bones)

TERM	DEFINITION
-pheresis	removal of blood from a donor with a portion separated and retained and the remainder reinfused into the donor; apheresis
-phoresis	indicating transmission (*as in* electrophoresis—transmission of electricity to separate substances)
pleural	pertaining to pleura
plural	more than one
pleuritis	inflammation of the pleura
pruritus	itching
prostate	gland at the base of the urinary bladder in males
prostrate	in a horizontal position; lying down
prostatic	pertaining to the prostate gland
prosthetic	pertaining to an artificial device or prosthesis (replacement of a body part)
-ptosis	droop, sag, prolapse
-ptysis	spitting
py/o	pus
pylor/o	pylorus (distal end of the stomach)
sacr/o	sacrum
sarc/o	flesh tissue
sclerosis	hardening
stenosis	narrowing
symphysis	fusion between two bones
synthesis	combining two parts to make something new

TERM	DEFINITION
ureter	one of two tubes each leading from a kidney to the urinary bladder
urethra	tube leading from the urinary bladder to the outside of the body
uvula	small, grape-like structure hanging from soft palate
vulva	external female genitalia
valvul/o	valve
volvulus	abnormal twisting of the intestine
vesical	pertaining to the urinary bladder
vesicle	a small blister

Specialized Terms Used in Medical Records*

The American Health Information Management Association has identified a group of terms used to compile statistical health care data and has defined them in an attempt at standardization. Some of these terms are presented in the following list, to highlight the importance of using standardized terms for research initiatives and the reporting of statistical data. The definitions are essentially those used by the American Health Information Management Association (some of the terms have multiple meanings, not provided here). *A Glossary of Health Care Terms*, a complete list of terms and definitions used in medical records, is available from the American Health Information Management Association, 919 N. Michigan Ave., Suite 1400, Chicago, IL 60611.

DIAGNOSIS: A word or phrase used by a physician to identify a disease from which an individual patient suffers or a condition for which a patient needs, seeks, or receives medical care.

PRINCIPAL DIAGNOSIS: The diagnosis of the condition established after study, chiefly responsible for occasioning the admission of the patient to the hospital for care.

OTHER DIAGNOSIS: A diagnosis, other than the principal diagnosis, that describes a condition for which a patient receives treatment or which the physician considers of sufficient significance to warrant inclusion for investigative medical studies.

COMPLICATION: An additional diagnosis that describes a condition arising after the beginning of hospital

*From Miller-Keane Encyclopedia & Dictionary of Medicine, Nursing, & Allied Health, 7th ed., revised reprint. Philadelphia, Saunders, 2005.

observation and treatment and modifying the course of the patient's illness or the medical care required.

MOST SIGNIFICANT DIAGNOSIS: The one diagnosis, often but not necessarily the principal diagnosis, that describes the most important or significant condition of a patient in terms of its implications for his or her health, medical care, and use of the hospital.

DISCHARGE DIAGNOSIS: Any one of the diagnoses recorded after all data accumulated in the course of a patient's hospitalization or other circumscribed episode of medical care have been studied.

DISCHARGE DIAGNOSES (LIST OF DISCHARGE DIAGNOSES): The complete set or list of discharge diagnoses applicable to a single patient experience such as inpatient hospitalization.

FACILITY: Those objects, including plant, equipment, or supplies, necessary for implementation of services by personnel.

HOSPITAL: Health care institution with an organized and professional staff and with inpatient beds available around the clock, whose primary function is to provide inpatient medical, nursing, and other health-related services to patients for both surgical and nonsurgical conditions, and that usually provides some outpatient services, particularly emergency care; for licensure purposes, each state has its own definition of "hospital."

HOSPITAL NEWBORN INPATIENT: A hospital patient who was born in the hospital at the beginning of his or her current inpatient hospitalization.

HOSPITAL BOARDER: An individual who receives lodging in the hospital but is not a hospital inpatient.

HOSPITAL INPATIENT BEDS: Accommodations with supporting services (such as food, laundry, and housekeeping) for hospital inpatients, excluding those for the newborn nursery.

HOSPITAL NEWBORN BASSINETS: Accommodations with supporting services (such as food, laundry, and housekeeping) for hospital newborn inpatients. These include bassinets, incubators, and Isolettes in the newborn nursery.

MEDICAL SERVICES: The activities related to medical care performed by physicians, nurses, and other professional and technical personnel under the direction of a physician.

OPERATING ROOM: An area of a hospital equipped and staffed to provide facilities and personnel services for the performance of surgical procedures.

DELIVERY ROOM: A special operating room for obstetric delivery and infant resuscitation.

UNIT: An organizational entity of a hospital. Hospitals are organized both physically and functionally into units.

MEDICAL STAFF UNIT: One of the departments, divisions, or specialties into which the organized medical staff of a hospital is divided in order to fulfill medical staff responsibility.

MEDICAL CARE UNIT: An assemblage of inpatient beds (or newborn bassinets) and related facilities and assigned personnel in which medical services are provided to a defined and limited class of patients according to their particular medical care needs.

HOSPITAL PATIENT: An individual receiving, in person, hospital-based or -coordinated medical services for which the hospital is responsible.

HOSPITAL INPATIENT: A hospital patient who is provided with room, board, and continuous general nursing service in an area of the hospital where patients generally stay at least overnight.

SPECIAL CARE UNIT: A medical care unit in which there is appropriate equipment and a concentration of physicians, nurses, and others who have special skills and experience to provide optimal medical care for critically ill patients, or continuous care of patients in special diagnostic categories.

ADJUNCT DIAGNOSTIC OR THERAPEUTIC UNIT (ANCILLARY UNIT): An organized unit of a hospital, other than the operating room, delivery room, or medical care unit, with facilities and personnel to aid physicians in the diagnosis and treatment of patients through the performance of diagnostic or therapeutic procedures.

Definitions of Diagnostic Tests and Procedures*

RADIOLOGY, ULTRASOUND, AND OTHER IMAGING PROCEDURES

In many of the following procedures, a *contrast* substance (sometimes referred to as a *dye*) is introduced into or around a body part so that the part can be better seen on x-ray images. The contrast substance (often containing barium or iodine) appears dense on the x-ray film and outlines the body part or tissue that it enters.

The suffix -GRAPHY, meaning "process of recording," is used in many terms describing imaging procedures. The suffix -GRAM, meaning "a record," is also used and usually describes the actual image that is produced by this procedure.

In the pronunciations provided for the listed terms, the syllable that gets the accent is in CAPITAL LETTERS. *Italicized* terms indicate important additional terminology, and terms in CAPITAL LETTERS are defined elsewhere in this listing.

ANGIOGRAPHY (an-je-OG-rah-fe) OR ANGIOGRAM (AN-je-o-gram): X-ray imaging of blood vessels. A contrast substance is injected into blood vessels (veins and arteries), and x-ray images are taken of the vessels. In *cerebral angiography*, x-ray images show blood vessels in the brain. In *coronary angiography*, x-rays detect abnormalities in vessels that bring blood to the heart. Angiograms can detect blockage by clots, cholesterol plaques, or tumors or aneurysms (ballooned or dilated areas of the vessel wall). Angiography is performed most frequently

---

*From Chabner DE: Medical Terminology: A Short Course, 5th ed. Philadelphia, Saunders, 2009.

to view arteries, so this term is often used interchangeably with *arteriography*.

ARTERIOGRAPHY (ar-te-re-OG-rah-fe) OR ARTE-RIOGRAM (ar-TE-re-oh-gram): X-ray imaging of arteries after injection of a contrast substance into an artery. *Coronary arteriography* is the visualization of arteries that travel across the outer surface of the heart and bring blood to the heart muscle.

ARTHROGRAPHY (arth-ROG-ra-fe): X-ray examination of the inside of a joint after instillation of a contrast medium.

BARIUM ENEMA: See LOWER GASTROINTESTINAL EXAMINATION and BARIUM TESTS.

BARIUM SWALLOW: See ESOPHAGOGRAPHY, BARIUM TESTS, and UPPER GASTROINTESTINAL EXAMINATION.

BARIUM TESTS (BAH-re-um TESTS): X-ray examinations performed with ingested liquid barium for contrast to locate disorders in the esophagus *(esophagogram)*, duodenum, small intestine *(small bowel follow-through)*, and colon *(barium enema)*. Ingested before or during the examination, barium causes the intestinal tract to stand out in silhouette when viewed through a *fluoroscope* or seen on an x-ray film. The *barium swallow* is used to examine the upper gastrointestinal tract, and the *barium enema* is for examination of the lower gastrointestinal tract.

BONE DENSITY SCAN (bon-DEN-se-te skan): Low-energy x-rays reveal areas of bone deficiency *(osteopenia)* and *osteoporosis* (bones become thinner, more fragile, and likely to break). It is most often performed on the lower spine or hips. Also called *bone densitometry* or *DEXA* (dual-energy x-ray absorptiometry).

CARDIAC CATHETERIZATION (KAR-de-ak cath-eh-ter-i-ZA-shun): Procedure in which a catheter (tube) is passed via vein or artery into the chambers of the heart to measure the blood flow out of the heart and the pressures and oxygen content in the heart chambers. Contrast material is also introduced into heart chambers, and x-ray images are taken to show heart structure.

CEREBRAL ANGIOGRAPHY: See ANGIOGRAPHY.

CHEST X-RAY (CHEST FILM OR RADIOGRAPH): An x-ray image of the chest wall, lungs, and heart. It may show infection (as in pneumonia or tuberculosis), emphysema, occupational exposure (asbestosis), lung tumors, or heart enlargement.

CHOLANGIOGRAPHY (kol-an-je-OG-rah-fe) OR CHOL-ANGIOGRAM (kol-AN-je-o-gram): X-ray imaging of bile ducts. Contrast material is given by intravenous injection *(IV cholangiogram)* and collects in the gallbladder and bile ducts. Also, contrast can be introduced (through the skin) with a percutaneously placed needle inserted into an intrahepatic duct *(percutaneous transhepatic cholangiography)*. X-rays are taken of bile ducts to identify obstructions caused by tumors or stones.

COMPUTED TOMOGRAPHY (CT) (kom-PU-ted to-MOG-ra-fe): X-ray imaging of the body in cross section. Contrast material may be used (injected into the bloodstream) to highlight structures such as the liver, brain, or blood vessels, and barium can be swallowed to outline gastrointestinal organs. X-ray images obtained as the x-ray tube rotates (helical CT) around the body are processed by a computer to show "slices" of body tissues, most often within the head, chest, and abdomen. (Sometimes called *CAT scan.*)

CORONARY ARTERIOGRAPHY: See ARTERIOGRAPHY.

CYSTOGRAPHY (sis-TOG-rah-fe) OR CYSTOGRAM (SIS-to-gram): X-ray imaging of the urinary bladder with a contrast medium so that the outline of the urinary bladder can be seen clearly. A contrast substance is injected through a catheter into the urethra and urinary bladder, and x-ray pictures are taken. A *voiding cystourethrogram* is an x-ray image of the urinary tract made while the patient is urinating.

DIGITAL SUBTRACTION ANGIOGRAPHY (DIJ-i-tal sub-TRAK-shun an-je-OG-rah-fe): A unique x-ray technique for viewing blood vessels by taking two images and "subtracting" one from the other. Images are first taken without contrast and then again after contrast is injected into blood vessels. The less-defined features on the first image are then subtracted from the second so that the final image (sharp and precise) shows only contrast-filled blood vessels and not the surrounding tissue.

DOPPLER ULTRASOUND (DOP-ler UL-tra-sound): Technique that focuses sound waves on blood vessels and measures blood flow as echoes bounce off red blood cells. Arteries or veins in the arms, neck, legs and abdomen are examined to detect vessels that are occluded (blocked) by clots or atherosclerosis.

ECHOCARDIOGRAPHY (eh-ko-kar-de-OG-rah-fe) OR ECHOCARDIOGRAM (eh-ko-KAR-de-o-gram): Images of the heart produced by directing high-frequency sound waves through the chest into the heart. The sound waves are reflected back from the heart, and echoes showing heart structure are displayed on a recording machine. It is a highly useful diagnostic tool in the evaluation of diseases of the valves that separate the heart chambers and diseases of the heart muscle.

ENDOSCOPIC RETROGRADE CHOLANGIOPAN-CREATOGRAPHY OR ERCP (en-do-SKOP-ik REH-tro-grad kol-an-je-o-pan-kre-ah-TOG-rah-fe): X-ray imaging of the bile ducts, pancreas, and pancreatic duct. Radiopaque contrast is injected via a tube through the mouth into the bile and pancreatic ducts, and x-ray pictures are then taken.

ENDOSCOPIC ULTRASONOGRAPHY OR E-US (en-do-SKOP-ik ul-trah-so-NOG-rah-fe): Sound waves are generated from a tube inserted through the mouth and into the esophagus. The sound waves bounce off of internal structures and are detected by surface coils. E-US detects enlarged lymph nodes and tumors in the chest and upper abdomen.

ESOPHAGOGRAPHY (eh-sof-ah-GOG-rah-fe) OR ESOPHAGOGRAM (eh-SOF-ah-go-gram): X-ray images taken of the esophagus after barium sulfate is swallowed. This test is part of a BARIUM SWALLOW and UPPER GASTROINTESTINAL EXAMINATION.

FLUOROSCOPY (flur-OS-ko-pe): An x-ray imaging procedure that uses a fluorescent screen rather than a photographic plate to show images of the body in motion. X-rays that have passed through the body strike a screen covered with a fluorescent substance that emits yellow-green light. Internal organs are seen directly (still images are stored either on film or on a computer as a digital image) and in motion. Fluoroscopy is used to guide the insertion of catheters for direct organ biopsy and may be enhanced with barium ingested by the patient.

GALLBLADDER ULTRASOUND (GAWL-blah-der UL-tra-sownd): Sound waves are used to visualize gallstones. This procedure has replaced the x-ray test *cholecystography.*

HYSTEROSALPINGOGRAPHY (his-ter-o-sal-ping-OG-rah-fe) OR HYSTEROSALPINGOGRAM (his-ter-o-sal-PING-o-gram): X-ray imaging of the uterus and fallopian tubes. Contrast medium is inserted through the vagina into the uterus and fallopian tubes, and x-ray pictures are taken to detect blockage or tumor.

INTRAVENOUS PYELOGRAPHY: See UROGRAPHY.

KIDNEYS, URETERS, BLADDER (KID-nez, UR-eh-terz, BLA-der) or KUB: X-ray images of the kidney, ureters, and urinary bladder, taken without contrast.

LOWER GASTROINTESTINAL EXAMINATION (LO-wer gas-tro-in-TES-tin-al ek-zam-ih-NA-shun): X-ray imaging of the colon taken after a liquid contrast substance called barium sulfate is inserted through a plastic tube (enema) into the rectum and large intestine (colon). If tumor is present in the colon, it may appear as an obstruction or irregularity. Also known as a BARIUM ENEMA.

MAGNETIC RESONANCE IMAGING (mag-NET-ik REZ-o-nans IM-a-jing) OR MRI: A powerful magnetic field, radio waves, and a computer produce detailed images of body organs. The images show several planes of the body—frontal (coronal), sagittal (side), and transverse (axial or cross-section)—and are particularly useful for studying tumors of the brain and spinal cord and abnormalities of the chest, abdomen, and head. No x-rays are used and MRI may be performed with or without contrast material. In *magnetic resonance angiography* (*MRA* or *MR angiography*), blood vessels are examined in key areas of the body such as the brain, kidneys, pelvis, legs, lung, and heart.

MAMMOGRAPHY (mah-MOG-rah-fe) OR MAMMO-GRAM (MAM-o-gram): X-ray imaging of the breast. X-rays of low voltage are beamed at the breast, and images are produced. Mammography detects abnormalities in breast tissue, such as breast cancer. In a *stereotactic breast biopsy*, a hollow needle is passed through the skin into a suspicious lesion with the help of mammography. A specialized mammography machine uses intersecting coordinates to pinpoint an area of tissue change (lesion).

MYELOGRAPHY (mi-eh-LOG-rah-fe) OR MYELOGRAM (MI-eh-lo-gram): X-ray imaging of the spinal cord. This procedure has been largely replaced by MRI to detect tumors or ruptured "slipped" disks between vertebrae (backbones).

PULMONARY ANGIOGRAPHY (PUL-mo-ner-e an-je-OG-rah-fe): X-ray imaging of blood vessels of the lung after injection of intravenous contrast.

PYELOGRAPHY OR PYELOGRAM: See UROGRAPHY.

SMALL BOWEL FOLLOW-THROUGH: See BARIUM TESTS and UPPER GASTROINTESTINAL EXAMINATION.

SONOGRAPHY: See ULTRASONOGRAPHY

TOMOGRAPHY (to-MOG-rah-fe) OR TOMOGRAM (TO-mo-gram): X-ray imaging that shows an organ in depth. Several pictures ("slices") are taken of an organ by moving the x-ray tube and film in sequence to blur out certain regions and bring others into sharper focus. Tomograms of the kidney and lung are examples.

ULTRASONOGRAPHY (ul-trah-so-NOG-rah-fe) OR ULTRASOUND (ul-trah-SOUND)/ULTRASOUND EXAMINATION: Images produced by beaming sound waves (not x-rays) into the body and capturing the echoes that bounce off organs. These echoes are then processed to produce an image showing the difference between fluid and solid masses and the general position of organs. Because ultrasound images are captured in real-time, they can show structure and movement of internal organs as well as blood flowing through blood vessels. Ultrasonography is particularly useful for detecting gallbladder stones, fibroid tumors of the uterus and ovarian tumors and cysts *(pelvic ultrasonography),* enlargement of the heart or defects in heart valves *(echocardiography),* blood flow through major arteries and veins (*Doppler ultrasound*), and enlargement of lymph nodes in the abdomen and chest. Also called *sonography.*

UPPER GASTROINTESTINAL EXAMINATION (UP-er gas-tro-in-TES-tin-al ek-zam-ih-NA-shun): X-ray imaging of the esophagus (BARIUM SWALLOW), duodenum, and small intestine after a liquid contrast substance (barium sulfate) is swallowed. In a *small bowel follow-through*, pictures are taken at increasing time intervals to follow the progress of barium through the small intestine. Identification of obstructions or ulcers is possible.

UROGRAPHY (u-ROG-rah-fe) OR UROGRAM (UR-o-gram): X-ray imaging of the kidney and urinary tract. If x-ray pictures are taken after contrast medium is injected intravenously, the procedure is called *intravenous urography* (*descending* or *excretion urography*) or *intravenous pyelography (IVP).* If the x-ray pictures are taken after instillation of contrast medium into the bladder through the urethra, the procedure is *retrograde urography* or *retrograde pyelography.* PYEL/O- means renal pelvis (the collecting chamber of the kidney).

NUCLEAR MEDICINE SCANS

In the following diagnostic tests, radioactive material *(radioisotope)* is injected intravenously or inhaled, and detected with a scanning device in the organ in which it accumulates. X-rays, ultrasound, or magnetic waves are not used.

BONE SCAN: A radioactive substance is injected intravenously, and its uptake in bones is detected with a scanning device. Tumors in bone can be detected by increased uptake of the radioactive material in the areas of the lesions.

BRAIN SCAN: A radioactive substance is injected intravenously. It collects in any lesion that disturbs the natural barrier that exists between blood vessels and normal brain tissue (blood-brain barrier), allowing the radioactive substance to enter the brain tissue. A scanning device detects the presence of the radioactive substance, which allows identification of an area of tumor, abscess, or hematoma.

GALLIUM SCAN (GAL-le-um skan): Radioactive gallium (gallium citrate) is injected into the bloodstream and is detected in the body with a scanning device that produces an image of the areas where gallium collects. The gallium collects in areas of certain tumors (as in Hodgkin disease) and in areas of infection.

MUGA SCAN (MUH-gah skan): Test that uses radioactive technetium to measure cardiac output. Also called *technetium-99m ventriculography* or *multiple-gated acquisition* scan.

POSITRON EMISSION TOMOGRAPHY (POS-i-tron e-MISH-un to-MOG-rah-fe) OR PET SCAN: Radioactive substances that release radioactive particles called positrons are injected into the body and travel to specialized areas of the body. Because of the way in which the positrons are released, cross-sectional color pictures can be made showing the location of the radioactive substance. The most common uses for PET scans are to detect cancer and to examine the effects of cancer therapy by showing biochemical changes in tumors. Tumors take up the radioactive substance (isotope) and appear as "hot spots" on the film. Also, PET scans can be performed on the heart to determine blood flow to heart muscle and evaluate coronary artery disease. PET scans of the brain are used to evaluate patients with memory disorders, seizure disorders, and brain tumors. *PET-CT* scans combine PET and CT imaging technology.

PULMONARY PERFUSION SCAN (PUL-mo-ner-e per-FU-shun skan): Radioactive particles are injected intravenously and travel rapidly to areas of the lung that are adequately filled with blood. Regions of obstructed blood flow caused by tumor, blood clot, swelling, and inflammation can be seen as nonradioactive areas on the scan.

PULMONARY VENTILATION SCAN (PUL-mo-ner-e ven-ti-LA-shun skan): Radioactive gas is inhaled, and a special camera detects its presence in the lungs. The scan is used to detect lung segments that fail to fill with the radioactive gas. Lack of filling is usually due to diseases that obstruct the bronchial tubes and air sacs. This scan is also used in the evaluation of lung function before surgery.

TECHNETIUM-99M SESTAMIBI SCAN (tek-NE-she-um 99m ses-ta-MIH-be skan): Technetium Tc 99m sestamibi is injected and taken up in areas of myocardial infarction (heart attack). This test can be used with an *exercise tolerance test (ETT-MIBI)* and is helpful in defining areas of decreased blood flow to heart muscle.

THALLIUM-201 SCINTIGRAPHY (THAL-e-um-201 SIN-tih-gra-fe): Thallium-201 is injected into a vein and images of blood flow through heart muscle are recorded. "Cold spots" (areas of little or no radioactivity) correlate with areas of restricted blood flow as from myocardial infarction. *Sestamibi scans (ETT-MIBI)* are also used to assess the status of blood flow through heart muscle during an exercise stress test.

THYROID SCAN AND UPTAKE (THI-royd skan and UP-take): In a thyroid scan, radioactive iodine (radiotracer) is injected intravenously or swallowed and collects in the thyroid gland. A scanning device (probe) detects the radiotracer in the gland, producing an image that shows the size, shape, and position of the thyroid gland. The radioactive iodine uptake (RAIU) test evaluates the function of the thyroid. Radioactive iodine is swallowed and a probe is placed over the thyroid gland to detect increased or decreased activity, which is shown by thyroid uptake of the radiotracer.

CLINICAL PROCEDURES

The following procedures are performed in patients to establish a correct diagnosis of an abnormal condition. In some instances, the procedure may also be used to treat the condition.

ABDOMINOCENTESIS (ab-dom-in-o-sen-TE-sis): See PARACENTESIS.

ALLERGY TEST (AL-er-je test): A small quantity of any of various suspected allergic substances is applied to the skin and a reaction is noted.

AMNIOCENTESIS (am-ne-o-sen-TE-sis): Surgical puncture to remove fluid from the sac (amnion) that surrounds the fetus in the uterus. The fluid contains cells from the fetus that can be examined with a microscope for chromosomal analysis. Levels of chemicals in amniotic fluid also can detect defects in the fetus.

ARTHROCENTESIS (ar-thro-sen-TE-sis): Surgical puncture to remove fluid from a joint.

ASPIRATION (as-peh-RA-shun): Withdrawal of fluid by suction through a needle or tube. The term *aspiration pneumonia* refers to an infection caused by inhalation into the lungs of food or an object.

AUDIOMETRY (aw-de-OM-eh-tre): Test using sound waves of various frequencies (e.g., 500 Hz) up to 8000 Hz, which quantifies the extent and type of hearing loss. An *audiogram* is the record produced by this test.

AUSCULTATION   (aw-skul-TA-shun): Process of listening for sounds produced within the body. This is most often performed with the aid of a stethoscope to determine the condition of the chest or abdominal organs or to detect the fetal heartbeat.

BIOPSY (BI-op-se): Removal of a piece of tissue from the body and subsequent examination of the tissue with a microscope. The procedure is performed with a surgical knife, by needle aspiration, or via endoscopic removal (using a special forceps-like instrument inserted through a hollow flexible tube.) An *excisional biopsy* means that the entire tissue to be examined is removed. An *incisional biopsy* is the removal of only a small amount of tissue, and a *needle biopsy* indicates that tissue is pierced with a hollow needle and fluid is withdrawn for microscopic examination.

BONE MARROW BIOPSY (bon MAH-ro BI-op-se): Removal of a small amount of bone marrow. The cells are then examined with a microscope. Often the hip bone (iliac crest) is used, and the biopsy is helpful in determining the number and type of blood cells in the bone marrow. Also called bone marrow aspiration.

BRONCHOSCOPY (brong-KOS-ko-pe): Insertion of a flexible tube (endoscope) into the airway. The lining of the bronchial tubes can be seen, and tissue may be removed for biopsy. The tube is usually inserted through the mouth but can also be directly inserted into the airway during mediastinoscopy. Sedation is required for this procedure.

CATHETERIZATION   (ka-ther-it-ih-ZA-shun): Introduction of a hollow, flexible tube into a vessel or cavity of the body to withdraw or instill fluids. Male and female *Foley catheters* are used for urinary catheterization. *Cardiac catheterization* involves insertion of a catheter into a large vein and threaded through the circulation system to the heart. Contrast can be administered to visualize blood vessels for diagnosis and treatment procedures.

CHORIONIC VILLUS SAMPLING (kor-e-ON-ik VIL-us SAM-pling): Removal and microscopic analysis of a small piece of placental tissue to detect fetal abnormalities.

COLONOSCOPY (ko-lon-OS-ko-pe): Insertion of a flexible tube (endoscope) through the rectum and into and upward through the colon for visual examination. Biopsy samples may be taken and benign growths, such as polyps, removed through the endoscope. The removal of a polyp is a *polypectomy* (pol-eh-PEK-to-me).

COLPOSCOPY (kol-POS-ko-pe): Inspection of the cervix through the insertion of a special microscope into the vagina. The vaginal walls are held apart with a speculum so that the cervix (entrance to the uterus) can come into view.

CONIZATION (ko-nih-ZA-shun): Removal of a cone-shaped sample of uterine cervix tissue. This sample is then examined with a microscope for evidence of cancerous growth. The special shape of the tissue sample allows the pathologist to examine the transitional zone of the cervix, where cancers are most likely to develop.

CULDOCENTESIS (kul-do-sen-TE-sis): Insertion of a thin, hollow needle through the vagina into the cul-de-sac, the space between the rectum and the uterus. Fluid is withdrawn and analyzed for evidence of cancerous cells, infection, or blood cells.

CYSTOSCOPY (sis-TOS-ko-pe): Insertion of a thin tube or cystoscope (endoscope) into the urethra and then into the urinary bladder to visualize the bladder and remove stones. A biopsy of the urinary bladder can be performed through the cystoscope.

DIGITAL RECTAL EXAMINATION (DIJ-ih-tal REK-tal eks-am-ih-NA-shun): A physician inserts a gloved finger into the rectum to detect rectal cancer and as a primary method to detect prostate cancer. The abbreviation is *DRE*.

DILATION AND CURETTAGE (di-LA-shun and kur-eh-TAJ): A series of probes of increasing size is systematically inserted through the vagina into the opening of the cervix. The cervix is thus dilated (widened) so that a curette (spoon-shaped instrument) can be inserted to remove tissue from the lining of the uterus. The tissue is then examined with a microscope. The abbreviation for this procedure is *D&C*.

ELECTROCARDIOGRAPHY   (e-lek-tro-kar-de-OG-rah-fe): Electrodes (wires or "leads") are connected to the body to record electrical impulses from the heart. The *electrocardiogram* is the actual record produced; it is useful in discovering abnormalities in heart rhythms and diagnosing heart disorders. The abbreviation is *ECG* (or *EKG*).

ELECTROENCEPHALOGRAPHY   (e-lek-tro-en-sef-ah-LOG-rah-fe): Connection of electrodes (wires or "leads") to the scalp to record electricity coming from within the brain. The electroencephalogram is the actual record produced. It is useful in the diagnosis and monitoring of epilepsy and other brain lesions and in the investigation of neurological disorders. It is also used to evaluate patients in coma (brain inactivity) and in the study of sleep disorders. The abbreviation is *EEG*.

ELECTROMYOGRAPHY   (e-lek-tro-mi-OG-rah-fe): Insertion of needle electrodes into muscle to record electrical activity. This procedure detects injuries and diseases that affect muscles and nerves. The abbreviation is *EMG*.

ENDOSCOPY (en-DOS-ko-pe): A thin, tube-like instrument (endoscope) is inserted into an organ or cavity to examine surrounding structures. The endoscope is placed through a natural opening (the mouth or anus) or into a surgical incision, such as through the abdominal wall. Endoscopes contain bundles of glass fibers that carry light (fiberoptic); some instruments are equipped with a small forceps-like device that withdraws a sample of tissue for microscopic study (biopsy). Examples of endoscopy are bronchoscopy, colonoscopy, esophagoscopy, gastroscopy, and laparoscopy.

ESOPHAGOGASTRODUODENOSCOPY (eh-SOF-ah-go-GAS-tro-du-o-de-NOS-ko-pe): An endoscope is inserted through the mouth and beyond to examine the esophagus, stomach, and first part of the small intestine. Also called *EGD*.

ESOPHAGOSCOPY (eh-sof-ah-GOS-ko-pe): An endoscope is inserted through the mouth and passed into the throat to examine the esophagus. This procedure permits detection of ulcers, tumors, or other lesions of the esophagus.

EXCISIONAL BIOPSY (ek-SIZH-in-al BI-op-se): See BIOPSY.

EXOPHTHALMOMETRY (eks-of-thal-MOM-eh-tre): Measurement of the extent of protrusion of the eyeball in *exophthalmos.*

FROZEN SECTION (fro-zen SEK-shun): Quick preparation of a biopsy sample for examination during an actual surgical procedure. Tissue is taken from the operating room to the pathology laboratory and frozen. It is then thinly sliced and immediately examined with a microscope to determine whether the sample is benign or malignant and to determine the status of margins.

GASTROSCOPY (gas-TROS-ko-pe): An endoscope is inserted through the esophagus and passed into the stomach for visual examination and/or biopsy of the stomach. When the upper portion of the small intestine is also visualized, the procedure is called *esophagogastroduodenoscopy (EGD)*

HOLTER MONITOR (HOL-ter MON-ih-ter): Electrocardiographic recording of heart activity over an extended period of time. The Holter monitor is worn by the patient as normal daily activities are performed. It detects and aids in the management of heart rhythm abnormalities. Also called *ambulatory electrocardiograph.*

HYSTEROSCOPY (his-ter-OS-ko-pe): An endoscope is inserted into the uterus for visual examination.

INCISIONAL BIOPSY (in-SIZH-in-al BI-op-se): See BIOPSY.

LAPAROSCOPY (lap-ah-ROS-ko-pe): Endoscopic examination of abdominal structures. After the patient receives a local anesthetic, a laparoscope is inserted through an incision in the abdominal wall. This procedure gives the physician a view of the abdominal cavity, the surface of the liver and spleen, and the pelvic region. A laparoscopic approach can be used instead of open surgery for removal of organs (such as the gallbladder, appendix, or ovary) and tumors, and for fallopian tube ligation to prevent pregnancy.

LARYNGOSCOPY (lah-rin-GOS-ko-pe): An endoscope is inserted into the airway to visually examine the voice box (larynx). A laryngoscope transmits a magnified image of the larynx through a system of lenses and mirrors. The procedure can reveal tumors and explain changes in the voice. Sputum samples and tissue biopsies are obtained by using brushes or forceps attached to the laryngoscope.

LUMBAR PUNCTURE (LUM-bar PUNK-shur): Introduction of a hollow needle into a space surrounding the spinal cord to withdraw fluid for analysis. The abbreviation is *LP*.

MEDIASTINOSCOPY (me-de-ah-sti-NOS-ko-pe): Insertion of an endoscope into the mediastinum (space in the chest between the lungs and in front of the heart). A mediastinoscope is inserted through a small incision in the neck while the patient is under anesthesia. This procedure is used to biopsy lymph nodes and to examine other structures within the mediastinum.

MUSCLE BIOPSY (MUS-el BI-op-se): A sample of muscle tissue is removed and analyzed microscopically.

NASOGASTRIC INTUBATION (na-zo-GAS-trik in-tu-BA-shun): Insertion of a tube through the nose into the stomach to withdraw fluid for analysis or to give nutrition directly into the stomach.

NEEDLE BIOPSY (NE-dl BI-op-se): See BIOPSY.

OPHTHALMOSCOPY (of-thal-MOS-ko-pe): A physician uses an *ophthalmoscope* to look directly into the eye, evaluating the optic nerve, retina, and blood vessels in the back of the eye and the lens in the front of the eye for cataracts. In *fluorescein angiography,* contrast is injected intravenously and movement of blood in the back of the eye is observed with ophthalmoscopy.

OTOSCOPY (o-TOS-ko-pe): A physician uses an *otoscope* inserted into the ear canal to check for obstructions (e.g., wax), infection, fluid, and eardrum perforations or scarring.

PALPATION (pal-PA-shun): Examination by touch. This is a technique of manual physical examination by which a physician feels underlying tissues and organs through the skin.

PAP SMEAR (pap smer): A cotton swab or wooden spatula is inserted into the vagina to obtain a sample of cells from the outer surface of the cervix (neck of the uterus). The cells are then smeared on a glass slide, preserved, and sent to the laboratory for microscopic examination. This test for cervical cancer was developed and named after Dr. George Papanicolaou. Results are reported as a grade I to IV (I = normal, II = inflammatory, III = suspicious for malignant disease, IV = malignant disease).

PARACENTESIS (pah-rah-sen-TE-sis): Surgical puncture of the membrane surrounding the abdomen (peritoneum) to remove fluid from the abdominal cavity. Fluid is drained for analysis and to prevent its accumulation in the abdomen. Also known as *abdominocentesis.*

PELVIC EXAM (PEL-vik ek-ZAM): Physician examines female sex organs and checks the uterus and ovaries for enlargement, cysts, tumors, or abnormal bleeding. This is also known as an "internal exam."

PERCUSSION (per-KUSH-un): The technique of striking a part of the body with short, sharp taps of the fingers to determine the size, density, and position of the underlying parts by the sound obtained. Percussion is commonly used on the abdomen to examine the liver.

PHLEBOTOMY (fleh-BOT-to-me): Incision of a vein to remove samples of blood for analysis. Also called *venipuncture*.

PROCTOSIGMOIDOSCOPY (prok-to-sig-moy-DOS-ko-pe): Insertion of an endoscope through the anus to examine the first 10 to 12 inches of the rectum and colon. When the sigmoid colon is visualized with a longer endoscope, the procedure is called *sigmoidoscopy*. The procedure detects polyps, malignant tumors, and sources of bleeding.

PULMONARY FUNCTION TEST (PUL-mo-ner-e FUNG-shun test): Measurement of the air taken into and exhaled from the lungs by means of an instrument called a *spirometer*. The test may be abnormal in patients with asthma, chronic bronchitis, emphysema, and occupational exposures to asbestos, chemicals, and dusts.

SIGMOIDOSCOPY (sig-moy-DOS-ko-pe): See PROCTOSIGMOIDOSCOPY.

STOOL CULTURE (stool KUL-chur): Feces (stools) placed in a growth medium (culture) are analyzed microscopically for evidence of microorganisms (bacteria).

STRESS TEST (stress test): An electrocardiogram taken during exercise. It may reveal hidden heart disease or confirm the cause of cardiac symptoms.

THORACENTESIS (thor-ah-sen-TE-sis): Insertion of a needle into the chest to remove fluid from the space surrounding the lungs (pleural cavity). After injection of a local anesthetic, a hollow needle is placed through the skin and muscles of the back and into the space between the lungs and chest wall. Fluid is then withdrawn by applying suction. Excess fluid *(pleural effusion)* may be a sign of infection or malignant disease. This procedure is used to diagnose conditions, to drain a pleural effusion, or to reexpand a collapsed lung *(atelectasis)*.

THORACOSCOPY (tho-ra-KOS-ko-pe): Insertion of an endoscope through an incision in the chest to visually examine the surface of the lungs. VATS is *video-assisted thoracoscopy (or thorascopy).*

TUNING FORK TESTS (TOO-ning fork tests): Tests of hearing using a vibrating tuning fork of known frequency as a source of sound.

LABORATORY TESTS

The following laboratory tests are performed on samples of a patient's blood, *plasma* (fluid portion of the blood), *serum* (plasma minus clotting proteins and produced after blood has clotted), urine, feces, *sputum* (mucus coughed up from the lungs), *cerebrospinal fluid* (fluid within the spaces around the spinal cord and brain), and skin.

ACID PHOSPHATASE (AH-sid FOS-fah-tas): Measurement of the amount of an enzyme called *acid phosphatase* in serum. Enzyme levels are elevated in metastatic prostate cancer. Moderate elevations of this enzyme occur in diseases of bone and when breast cancer cells invade bone tissue.

ALBUMIN (al-BU-min): Measurement of the amount of albumin (protein) in both the serum and the urine. A decrease of albumin in serum indicates disease of the kidneys, malnutrition, or liver disease or may occur with extensive loss of protein in the gut or from the skin, as in a burn. The presence of albumin in the urine (*albuminuria*) indicates malfunction of the kidney.

ALKALINE PHOSPHATASE (AL-kah-lin FOS-fah-tays): Measurement of the amount of *alkaline phosphatase* (an enzyme found on cell membranes) in serum. Levels are elevated in liver diseases (such as hepatitis and hepatoma) and in bone disease and bone cancer. The laboratory abbreviation is *alk phos.*

ALPHA-FETOPROTEIN (al-fa-fe-to-PRO-teen): Determination of the presence of a protein called alpha-globulin in serum. The protein is normally present in the serum of the fetus, infant, and pregnant woman. In fetuses with abnormalities of the brain and spinal cord, the protein leaks into the amniotic fluid surrounding the fetus and is an indicator of spinal tube defect (spina bifida) or anencephaly (lack of brain development). High levels are found in patients with cancer of the liver and other malignant diseases (testicular and ovarian cancers). Serum levels monitor the effectiveness of cancer treatment. Elevated levels are also seen in benign liver disease such as cirrhosis and viral hepatitis. The laboratory abbreviation is *AFP.*

ALT: Measurement of the amount of the enzyme called *alanine transaminase* in serum. The enzyme is normally present in blood but accumulates in blood with damage to liver cells. Also called *SGPT.*

ANA: See ANTINUCLEAR ANTIBODY TEST.

ANTINUCLEAR ANTIBODY TEST (an-tih-NU-kle-ar AN-tih-bod-e test): A sample of plasma is tested for the presence of antibodies that are found in patients with systemic lupus erythematosus. Laboratory abbreviation is *ANA.*

AST: Measurement of the enzyme *aspartate transaminase* in serum. The enzyme is normally present in blood but accumulates when there is damage to the heart or to liver cells. Also called *SGOT.*

BACTERIAL AND FUNGAL TESTS (bak-TER-e-al and FUNG-al tests): Samples from skin lesions are analyzed microscopically to diagnose bacterial or fungal conditions.

BENCE JONES PROTEIN (bens jonz PRO-ten): Measurement of the presence of the Bence Jones protein in serum or urine. Bence Jones protein is a fragment of a normal serum protein, an immunoglobulin, produced by cancerous bone marrow cells (myeloma cells). Normally it is not found in either blood or urine, but in *multiple myeloma* (a malignant condition of bone marrow), high levels of Bence Jones protein are detected in urine and serum.

BILIRUBIN (bil-ih-RU-bin): Measurement of the amount of bilirubin, an orange-brown pigment, in serum and urine. Bilirubin is derived from hemoglobin, the oxygen-carrying protein in red blood cells. Its presence in high concentration in serum and urine causes *jaundice* (yellow coloration of the skin) and may indicate disease of the liver, obstruction of bile ducts, or a type of anemia that leads to excessive destruction of red blood cells.

BLOOD CHEMISTRY PROFILE: A comprehensive blood test that is a biochemical examination of various substances in the blood using a computerized laboratory analyzer. Tests include calcium (bones), phosphorus (bones), urea (kidney), creatinine (kidney), bilirubin (liver), AST (liver and heart muscle) and ALT (liver), alkaline phosphatase (liver and bone), globulin (liver and immune disorders), and albumin (liver and kidney). Also called SMA or sequential multiple analysis. SMA-6, SMA-12, and SMA-18 indicate the number of blood elements tested.

BLOOD CULTURE (blud KUL-chur): Test to determine whether infection is present in the bloodstream. A sample of blood is added to a special medium (food) that promotes the growth of microorganisms. The medium is then examined by a medical technologist for evidence of bacteria or other microbes.

BLOOD UREA NITROGEN (blud u-RE-ah NI-tro-jen): Measurement of the amount of urea (nitrogen-containing waste material) in serum. A high level of serum urea indicates poor kidney function because it is the kidney's job to remove urea from the bloodstream and filter it into urine. The laboratory abbreviation is *BUN*.

CA-125: Protein released into the bloodstream by ovarian cancer cells. Measurement of CA-125 determines response to treatment.

CALCIUM (KAL-se-um): Measurement of the amount of calcium in serum, plasma, or whole blood. Low blood levels are associated with abnormal functioning of nerves and muscles, and high blood levels indicate loss of calcium from bones, excessive intake of calcium, disease of the parathyroid glands, or cancer. The laboratory symbol for calcium is *Ca.*

CARBON DIOXIDE (KAR-bon di-OK-side): Blood test to measure the gas produced in tissues and eliminated by the lungs. Abnormal levels may reflect lung disorders. The laboratory symbol for carbon dioxide is CO_2.

CARCINOEMBRYONIC ANTIGEN (kar-sih-no-em-bree-ON-ik AN-ti-jen): A plasma test for a protein normally found in the blood of human fetuses and produced in healthy adults only in a very small amount, if at all. High levels of this antigen may be a sign of one of a variety of cancers, especially colon or pancreatic cancer. This test monitors the response of patients to cancer treatment. The laboratory abbreviation is *CEA.*

CEREBROSPINAL FLUID (seh-re-bro-SPI-nal FLU-id): Measurement of cerebrospinal fluid for protein, sugar, and blood cells. The fluid is also cultured to detect microorganisms. Chemical tests are performed on specimens of the fluid removed by *lumbar puncture.* Abnormal conditions such as meningitis, brain tumor, and encephalitis are detected. The laboratory abbreviation is *CSF.*

CHOLESTEROL (ko-LES-ter-ol): Measurement of the amount of cholesterol (substance found in animal fats and oils, egg yolks, and milk) in serum or plasma. Normal values vary for age and diet; levels above 200 mg/dl indicate a need for further testing and efforts to reduce cholesterol level because high levels are associated with hardening of arteries and heart disease. Blood is also tested for the presence of a lipoprotein substance that is a combination of cholesterol and protein. High levels (optimum level is 60 to 100 mg/dL) of high-density lipoprotein (*HDL*) cholesterol in the blood are beneficial because HDL cholesterol promotes the removal and excretion of excess cholesterol from the body, whereas high levels of low-density lipoprotein *(LDL)* are associated with the development of atherosclerosis (optimum level is 100 mg/dL or less).

COMPLETE BLOOD COUNT (CBC): Determinations of the numbers of leukocytes (white blood cells), erythrocytes (red blood cells), and platelets (clotting cells). The CBC is useful in diagnosis of anemia, infection, and blood cell disorders, such as leukemia.

CREATINE KINASE (KRE-ah-tin KI-nays): Measurement of levels of creatine kinase, a blood enzyme. Creatine kinase is normally found in heart muscle, brain tissue, and skeletal muscle. The presence of one form *(isoenzyme)* of creatine kinase (either CK-MB or CK2) in the blood is strongly indicative of recent myocardial infarction (heart attack) because the enzyme is released from heart muscle when the muscle is damaged or dying.

CREATININE (kre-AT-tih-nin): Measurement of the amount of creatinine, a nitrogen-containing waste material, in serum or plasma. It is the most reliable test for kidney function. Because creatinine is normally produced as a protein breakdown product in muscle and is excreted by the kidney in urine, an elevation in the creatinine level in the blood indicates a disturbance of kidney function. Elevations are also seen in high-protein diets and dehydration.

CREATININE CLEARANCE (kre-AT-tih-nin KLER-ans): Measurement of the rate at which creatinine is cleared (filtered) by the kidneys from the blood. A low creatinine clearance indicates that the kidneys are not functioning effectively to clear creatinine from the bloodstream and filter it into urine.

CULTURE (KUL-chur): Identification of microorganisms grown in a special laboratory medium (fluid, solid, or semisolid material). In *sensitivity* tests, culture plates containing a specific microorganism are prepared and antibiotic-containing disks are applied to the culture surface. After overnight incubation, the area surrounding the disk (where growth was inhibited) is measured to determine whether the antibiotic is effective against the specific organism.

DIFFERENTIAL (di-fer-EN-shul): See WHITE BLOOD CELL COUNT.

ELECTROLYTES (e-LEK-tro-litz): Determination of the concentration of different *electrolytes* (chemical substances capable of conducting an electric current) in serum or whole blood. When dissolved in water, electrolytes break apart into charged particles *(ions)*. The positively charged electrolytes are *sodium* (Na^+), *potassium* (K^+), *calcium* (Ca^{2+}), and *magnesium* (Mg^{2+}). The negatively charged electrolytes are *chloride* (Cl^-) and *bicarbonate* (HCO_3^-). These charged particles should be present at all times for proper functioning of cells. An electrolyte imbalance occurs when serum concentration is either too high or too low. Calcium balance can affect the bones, kidneys, gastrointestinal tract, and neuromuscular activity, and sodium balance affects blood pressure, nerve functioning, and fluid levels surrounding cells. Potassium balance affects heart and muscular activity.

ELECTROPHORESIS: See SERUM PROTEIN ELECTROPHORESIS.

ELISA (eh-LI-zah): A laboratory assay (test) for the presence of antibodies to the AIDS virus. A positive result indicates a high likelihood that the patient's blood contains the AIDS virus (HIV or human immunodeficiency virus). The presence of the virus stimulates white blood cells to make antibodies that are detected by the ELISA assay. This is the first test done to detect AIDS infection and is followed by a Western blot test to confirm the results. ELISA is an acronym for *enzyme-l*inked *i*mmun*o*sorbent *a*ssay.

ERYTHROCYTE SEDIMENTATION RATE (eh-RITH-ro-sit sed-ih-men-TA-shun rat): Measurement of the rate at which red blood cells (erythrocytes) in well-mixed venous blood settle to the bottom (sediment) of a test tube. If the rate of sedimentation is markedly slow (elevated sed rate), it may indicate inflammatory conditions, such as rheumatoid arthritis, or conditions that produce excessive proteins in the blood. Laboratory abbreviations are *ESR* and *sed rate*.

ESTRADIOL (es-tra-DI-ol): Test for the concentration of estradiol, which is a form of estrogen (female hormone) in serum, plasma, or urine.

ESTROGEN RECEPTOR ASSAY (ES-tro-jen re-SEP-tor AS-a): Test, performed at the time of a biopsy, to determine whether a sample of tumor contains an estrogen receptor protein. The protein, if present on breast cancer cells, combines with estrogen, allowing estrogen to promote the growth of the tumor. Thus if an estrogen receptor assay result is positive (the protein is present), then treatment with an antiestrogen drug would retard tumor growth. If the assay is negative (the protein is not present), then the tumor would not be affected by antiestrogen drug treatment.

GLOBULIN (GLOB-u-lin): Measurement (in serum) of proteins that bind to and destroy foreign substances (antigens). Globulins are made by cells of the immune system. *Gamma globulin* is one type of globulin that contains antibodies to fight disease.

GLUCOSE (GLU-kos): Measurement of the amount of glucose (sugar) in serum and plasma. High levels of glucose *(hyperglycemia)* indicate diseases such as diabetes mellitus and hyperthyroidism. Glucose is also measured in urine, and its presence indicates diabetes mellitus. *Fasting blood sugar test* is measurement of blood sugar after a patient has fasted.

GLUCOSE TOLERANCE TEST (GLU-kos TOL-er-ans test): Test to determine how the body uses glucose. In the first part of this test, blood and urine samples are taken after the patient has fasted. Then a solution of glucose is given by mouth. A half hour after the glucose is taken, blood and urine samples are obtained again and are collected every hour for 4 to 5 hours. This test can indicate abnormal conditions such as diabetes mellitus, hypoglycemia, and liver or adrenal gland dysfunction.

HEMATOCRIT (he-MAT-o-krit): Measurement of the percentage of blood volume occupied by red blood cells. The normal range is 40% to 50% in males and 37% to 47% in females. A low hematocrit indicates anemia. The laboratory abbreviation is *Hct*.

HEMOCCULT TEST (he-mo-KULT test): Examination of small sample of stool for otherwise inapparent occult (hidden) traces of blood. The sample is placed on the surface of a collection kit and reacts with a chemical (e.g., guaiac). A positive result may indicate bleeding from polyps, ulcers, or malignant tumors. This is an important screening test for colon cancer. Also called a STOOL GUAIAC TEST.

HEMOGLOBIN ASSAY (HE-mo-glo-bin AS-a): Measurement of the concentration of hemoglobin in blood. The normal blood hemoglobin ranges are 13.5 to 18.0 gm/dl in adult males and 12.0 to 16.0 gm/dl in adult females. The laboratory abbreviation is *Hgb*.

HUMAN CHORIONIC GONADOTROPIN (HU-man kor-e-ON-ik go-nad-o-TRO-pin): Measurement of the concentration of human chorionic gonadotropin (a hormone secreted by cells of the fetal placenta) in urine. It can be detected in urine within days after fertilization of egg and sperm cells; this is the basis for the most commonly used pregnancy test. The abbreviation is *hCG*.

IMMUNOASSAY (im-u-no-AS-a): A method of testing blood and urine for the concentration of various chemicals, such as hormones, drugs, or proteins. The technique makes use of the immunologic reaction between antigens and antibodies. An *assay* is a determination of the amount of any particular substance in fluid or tissue.

IMMUNOHISTOCHEMISTRY (im-u-no-his-to-KEM-is-tre): An antibody tagged with a radioactive or fluorescent label is spread over a tissue biopsy specimen and used to detect the presence of an antigen (protein) produced by the tissue or infection.

LIPID TESTS (LIP-id tests): Lipids are fatty substances such as cholesterol and triglycerides. See CHOLESTEROL and TRIGLYCERIDE.

LIPOPROTEIN TESTS (li-po-PRO-teen tests): See CHOLESTEROL.

LIVER FUNCTION TESTS (LIV-er FUNG-shun tests): See ALKALINE PHOSPHATASE, BILIRUBIN, ALT, and AST.

OCCULT BLOOD TEST: See HEMOCCULT TEST.

PKU TEST: Test that determines whether the urine of a newborn baby contains substances called *phenylketones*. If so, the condition is called *phenylketonuria (PKU)*. Phenylketonuria occurs in infants born lacking a specific enzyme. If the enzyme is missing, high levels of *phenylalanine* (an amino acid) accumulate in the blood, affecting the infant's brain and causing mental retardation. This situation is prevented by placing the infant on a special diet that prevents accumulation of phenylalanine in the bloodstream.

PLATELET COUNT (PLAT-let kownt): Determination of the number of clotting cells (platelets) in a sample of blood.

POTASSIUM (po-TAHS-e-um): Measurement of the concentration of potassium in serum. Potassium combines with other minerals (such as calcium) and is an important chemical for proper functioning of muscles, especially the heart muscle. The symbol for potassium is K^+. See also ELECTROLYTES.

PREGNANCY TEST (PREG-nan-se test): Measurement in blood or urine of *human chorionic gonadotropin* (hCG), a hormone secreted by the placenta early in pregnancy.

PROGESTERONE RECEPTOR ASSAY (pro-JES-teh-rone re-SEP-tor AS-a): Test to determines whether a sample of tumor contains a progesterone receptor protein. A positive test result indicates that the breast cancer tumor would be responsive to antihormone therapy.

PROSTATE-SPECIFIC ANTIGEN (PROS-tat spe-SIF-ic AN-ti-jen): Blood test that measures the amount of an antigen elevated in all patients with prostatic cancer and in some with an inflamed prostate gland. The laboratory abbreviation is *PSA*.

PROTEIN ELECTROPHORESIS: See SERUM PROTEIN ELECTROPHORESIS.

PROTHROMBIN TIME (pro-THROM-bin tim): Measurement of the activity of factors in the blood that participate in clotting. Deficiency of any of these factors can lead to a prolonged prothrombin time and difficulty in blood clotting. The test is important as a monitor for patients taking anticoagulants, substances that block the activity of blood clotting factors and increase the risk of bleeding.

PSA: See PROSTATE-SPECIFIC ANTIGEN.

RED BLOOD CELL (RBC) COUNT: Test in which the number of erythrocytes in a sample of blood is counted. A low red blood cell count may indicate anemia. A high count can indicate *polycythemia vera.*

RHEUMATOID FACTOR (ROO-mah-toyd FAK-tor): Detection of the abnormal protein *rheumatoid factor* in the serum. It is found in patients with rheumatoid arthritis.

SEMEN ANALYSIS (SE-men ah-NAL-ih-sis): Microscopic examination of sperm cells to detect viability and motility of sperm cells.

SERUM ENZYME TESTS (SE-rum EN-zim tests): Measurements of enzymes released into the bloodstream after a heart attack. Examples are creatine kinase (CK) and troponin I and troponin T.

SERUM AND URINE TESTS (SE-rum and UR-in tests): Measurements of hormones, electrolytes, and glucose among other substances as indicators of endocrine and other body functions.

SERUM PROTEIN ELECTROPHORESIS (SE-rum PRO-teen e-lek-tro-for-E-sis): A procedure that separates proteins with an electric current. The material tested, such as serum, containing various proteins, is placed on paper or gel or in liquid, and under the influence of an electric current, the proteins separate (-PHORESIS means separation) so that they can be identified and measured. The procedure is also known as *protein electrophoresis*.

SGOT: See AST.

SGPT: See ALT.

SKIN TESTS: Tests in which substances are applied to the skin or injected under the skin and the reaction of immune cells in the skin is observed. These tests detect a patient's sensitivity to substances such as dust or pollen. They can also indicate whether a patient has been exposed to the bacteria that cause tuberculosis or diphtheria.

SLIT-LAMP MICROSCOPY (slit-lamp mi-KROS-ko-pe): Microscopic examination of anterior eye structures.

SMA: See BLOOD CHEMISTRY PROFILE.

SODIUM: Measurement of the concentration of sodium in serum. Sodium is one of the most important elements in the body. It is the chief *electrolyte* in fluid outside cells and it interacts with potassium within cells. It is involved in water balance, acid-base chemical balance, nerve transmission, and contraction of muscles. The symbol for sodium is *Na*.

SPUTUM TEST (SPU-tum test): Examination of mucus coughed up from a patient's lungs to detect tumor or infection. The sputum is examined microscopically and chemically and is cultured for the presence of microorganisms.

STOOL GUAIAC TEST (stool GWI-ak test): See HEMOCCULT TEST.

THYROID FUNCTION TESTS (THI-royd FUNG-shun tests): Tests that measure the levels of thyroid hormones, such as *thyroxine* (T_4) and *triiodothyronine* (T_3), in serum. *Thyroid-stimulating hormone (TSH),* which is produced by the pituitary gland and stimulates the release of

T_4 and T_3 from the thyroid gland, is also measured in serum. These tests diagnose hypothyroidism and hyperthyroidism and are helpful in monitoring response to thyroid treatment.

TRIGLYCERIDE (tri-GLIS-er-ide): Determination of the amount of triglycerides (simple fats) in the serum. Elevated triglyceride levels (normal is 200 mg to 300 mg/dL) are considered an important risk factor for the development of heart disease.

TROPONIN (tro-PO-nin): Measurement of levels of proteins troponin I and troponin T in the bloodstream after myocardial injury (heart attack).

URIC ACID (UR-ik AS-id): Measurement of the amount of uric acid (a nitrogen-containing waste material) in the serum and urine. High serum levels indicate a type of arthritis called *gout*. In gout, uric acid accumulates as crystals in joints and in tissues. High levels of uric acid may also cause kidney stones.

URINALYSIS (u-rih-NAL-ih-sis): Examination of urine as an aid in the diagnosis of disease. Routine urinalysis involves the observation of unusual color or odor; determination of specific gravity (amount of materials dissolved in urine); chemical tests (for protein, sugar, acetone); and microscopic examination for bacteria, blood cells, and sediment. Urinalysis is used to detect abnormal functioning of the kidneys and bladder, infections, abnormal growths, and diabetes mellitus. The laboratory abbreviation is *UA.*

WESTERN BLOT (WES-tern blot): Test used to detect infection by *HIV* (AIDS virus). It is more specific than the ELISA. A patient's serum is mixed with purified proteins from HIV, and the reaction is examined. If the patient has made antibodies to HIV, those antibodies react with the purified HIV proteins and the test result is positive.

WHITE BLOOD CELL (WBC) COUNT: Determination of the number of leukocytes in the blood. Higher than normal counts can indicate the presence of infection or leukemia. A *differential* (or differential count) gives the percentages of different types of white blood cells (neutrophils, eosinophils, basophils, lymphocytes, and monocytes) in a sample of blood. It provides more specific information about leukocytes and aids in the diagnosis of infection, allergic diseases, disorders of the immune system, and various forms of leukemia.

PART 2

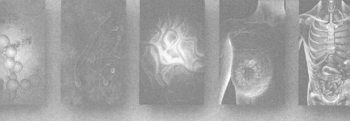

Useful Information

Abbreviations for Selected Health Care Organizations, Associations, and Agencies*

AAAA	American Academy of Anesthesiologist Assistants
AAAAI	American Academy of Allergy, Asthma, and Immunology
AAATP	Association for Anesthesiologist's Assistants Training Program
AAB	American Association of Bioanalysts
AABB	American Association of Blood Banks
AACA	American Association of Clinical Anatomists
AACAHPO	American Association of Certified Allied Health Personnel in Ophthalmology
AACC	American Association for Clinical Chemistry
AACN	American Association of Critical Care Nurses
	American Association of Colleges of Nursing
AACP	American Academy of Clinical Psychiatrists; American Association of Colleges of Pharmacy
AADS	American Association of Dental Schools
AHIMA	American Health Information Management Association
AAFP	American Academy of Family Physicians

---

*Modified from Miller-Keane Encyclopedia & Dictionary of Medicine, Nursing, & Allied Health, 7th ed., revised reprint. Philadelphia, WB Saunders, 2005.

**ABBREVIATIONS FOR SELECTED HEALTH CARE
ORGANIZATIONS, ASSOCIATIONS, AND AGENCIES**
(Continued)

AAHA	American Academy of Health Administration
AAHC	Association of Academic Health Centers
AAHE	Association for the Advancement of Health Education
AAHP	American Association of Health Plans
AAHPER	American Association for Health, Physical Education, and Recreation
AAMA	American Association of Medical Assistants
AAMC	Association of American Medical Colleges
AAMI	Association for the Advancement of Medical Instrumentation
AAMT	American Association for Music Therapy
AAN	American Academy of Neurology
	American Academy of Nursing
AANA	American Association of Nurse Anesthetists
AAO	American Association of Ophthalmology
	American Association of Orthodontists
AAOHN	American Association of Occupational Health Nurses
AAP	American Academy of Pediatrics
AAPA	American Academy of Physicians Assistants
AAPMR	American Academy of Physical Medicine and Rehabilitation
AARC	American Association for Respiratory Care
AART	American Association for Rehabilitation Therapy
AATA	American Art Therapy Association
AATS	American Association for Thoracic Surgery
ABCP	American Board of Cardiovascular Perfusion

**ABBREVIATIONS FOR SELECTED HEALTH CARE
ORGANIZATIONS, ASSOCIATIONS, AND AGENCIES**
(Continued)

ABNF	Association of Black Nursing Faculty in Higher Education
ACAAI	American College of Asthma, Allergy & Immunology
ACC	American College of Cardiology
ACCP	American College of Chest Physicians
ACEN	Academy of Canadian Executive Nurses
ACEP	American College of Emergency Physicians
ACHA	American College of Hospital Administrators
ACNM	American College of Nurse-Midwives
ACP	American College of Physicians
ACR	American College of Radiology
ACS	American College of Surgeons
ACTA	American Cardiovascular Technologists Association
ADA	American Dental Association
ADAA	American Dental Assistants Association
ADHA	American Dental Hygienists' Association
ADTA	American Dance Therapy Association
AES	American Electroencephalographic Society
AHA	American Hospital Association
AHCPR	Agency for Health Care Policy and Research [now AHRQ]
AHPA	American Health Planning Association
AHRQ	Agency for Healthcare Research and Quality
AIBS	American Institute of Biological Sciences
AIHA	American Industrial Hygiene Association
AIUM	American Institute of Ultrasound in Medicine

**ABBREVIATIONS FOR SELECTED HEALTH CARE
ORGANIZATIONS, ASSOCIATIONS, AND AGENCIES**
(Continued)

AMA	American Medical Association
AMEA	American Medical Electroencephalographic Association
AMI	Association of Medical Illustrators
AMIA	American Medical Informatics Association
AmSECT	American Society of Extra-Corporeal Technology
AMSN	Academy of Medical-Surgical Nurses
AMT	American Medical Technologists
ANA	American Nurses Association
ANCC	American Nurses Credentialing Center
ANF	American Nurses Foundation
ANHA	American Nursing Homes Association
ANNA	American Nephrology Nurses' Association
ANRC	American National Red Cross
AOA	American Optometric Association American Osteopathic Association
AONE	American Organization of Nurse Executives
AORN	Association of Operating Room Nurses
AOTA	American Occupational Therapy Association
APA	American Podiatry Association American Psychiatric Association American Psychological Association
APAP	Association of Physician Assistants Programs
APHA	American Public Health Association
APIC	Association of Practitioners in Infection Control
APTA	American Physical Therapy Association
ARCA	American Rehabilitation Counseling Association

**ABBREVIATIONS FOR SELECTED HEALTH CARE
ORGANIZATIONS, ASSOCIATIONS, AND AGENCIES**
(Continued)

ARN	Association of Rehabilitation Nurses
ASA	American Society of Anesthesiologists
ASAHP	American Society of Allied Health Professionals
ASC	American Society of Cytotechnology
ASCP	American Society of Clinical Pathologists
ASE	American Society of Echocardiography
ASET	American Society of Electroencephalographic Technologists
ASHA	American Speech-Language-Hearing Association
ASIA	American Spinal Injury Association
ASIM	American Society of Internal Medicine
ASM	American Society of Microbiology
ASMT	American Society for Medical Technology
ASNSA	American Society of Nursing Service Administrators
ASPAN	American Association of PeriAnesthesia Nurses
ASPH	Association of Schools of Public Health
ASRT	American Society of Radiologic Technologists
AST	Association of Surgical Technologists
ASUTS	American Society of Ultrasound Technical Specialists
ATS	American Thoracic Society
AUPHA	Association of University Programs in Health Administration
AVA	American Vocational Association
AVMA	American Veterinary Medical Association
CAAHEP	Committee on Accreditation of Allied Health Education Programs
CAN	Canadian Nurses Association

**ABBREVIATIONS FOR SELECTED HEALTH CARE
ORGANIZATIONS, ASSOCIATIONS, AND AGENCIES**
(Continued)

CAP	College of American Pathologists
CCHFA	Canadian Council of Health Facilities Accreditation
CCHSE	Canadian Council of Health Service Executives
CCNE	Commission on Collegiate Nursing Education
CDC	Centers for Disease Control and Prevention
CGFNS	Commission on Graduates of Foreign Nursing Schools
CGNA	Canadian Gerontological Nursing Association
CME (AMA)	Council on Medical Education of the American Medical Association
COEAMRA	Council on Education of the American Medical Record Association
DHHS	Department of Health and Human Services
ENA	Emergency Nurses Association
FDA	Food and Drug Administration
HCFA	Health Care Financing Administration
HRA	Health Resources Administration
HSCA	Health Sciences Communications Association
HSRA	Health Services and Resources Administration
IAET	International Association for Enterostomal Therapy
IOM	Institute of Medicine of the National Academy of Sciences
ISCVS	International Society for Cardiovascular Surgery
JCAHO	Joint Commission on the Accreditation of Healthcare Organizations
JCAHPO	Joint Commission on Allied Health Personnel in Ophthalmology

ABBREVIATIONS FOR SELECTED HEALTH CARE ORGANIZATIONS, ASSOCIATIONS, AND AGENCIES
(Continued)

MLA	Medical Library Association
NAACLS	National Accrediting Agency for Clinical Laboratory Science
NAACOG	Nurses Association of the American Association of Obstetrics and Gynecology
NACA	National Advisory Council on Aging (Canada)
NACCHO	National Association of County and City Health Officials
NACT	National Alliance of Cardiovascular Technologists
NADONA/ LTC	National Association of Directors of Nursing Administration in Long Term Care
NAEMT	National Association of Emergency Medical Technicians
NAHC	National Association of Home Care
NAHSR	National Association of Human Services Technologists
NAMT	National Association for Music Therapy
NANDA	North American Nursing Diagnosis Association
NANT	National Association of Nephrology Technologists
NAPNES	National Association for Practical Nurse Education and Services
NARF	National Association of Rehabilitation Facilities
NASMD	National Association of State Medical Directors
NASW	National Association of Social Workers
NATTS	National Association of Trade and Technical Schools
NBNA	National Black Nurses Association
NCEHPHP	National Council on the Education of Health Professionals in Health Promotion

ABBREVIATIONS FOR SELECTED HEALTH CARE
ORGANIZATIONS, ASSOCIATIONS, AND AGENCIES
(Continued)

NCHS	National Center for Health Statistics
NCRE	National Council on Rehabilitation Education
NEHA	National Environmental Health Education
NFLPN	National Federation of Licensed Practical Nurses
NHC	National Health Council
NHSC	National Health Services Corps
NIH	National Institutes of Health
NIOSH	National Institute of Occupational Safety and Health
NKF	National Kidney Foundation
NLN	National League for Nursing
NNBA	National Nurses in Business Association
NOLF	Nursing Organization Liaison Forum
NONPF	National Organization of Nurse Practitioner Faculties
NPWH	National Association of Nurse Practitioners in Women's Health
NRCA	National Rehabilitation Counseling Association
NREMT	National Registry of Emergency Medical Technicians
NSCPT	National Society for Cardiopulmonary Technology
NSH	National Society for Histotechnology
NSNA	National Student Nurses Association
NTRS	National Therapeutic Recreation Society
NTSAD	National Tay-Sachs and Allied Diseases Association
OAA	Opticians Association of America
ONS	Oncology Nurses Association
PNAA	Philippine Nurses Association of America

**ABBREVIATIONS FOR SELECTED HEALTH CARE
ORGANIZATIONS, ASSOCIATIONS, AND AGENCIES**
(Continued)

RWJF	The Robert Wood Johnson Foundation
SDMS	Society of Diagnostic Medical Sonographers
SNIVT	Society of Non-invasive Vascular Technology
SNM	Society of Nuclear Medicine
SNMTS	Society of Nuclear Medicine Technologist Section
SOPHE	Society for Public Health Education
STS	Society of Thoracic Surgeons
STTI	Sigma Theta Tau International
SVS	Society for Vascular Surgery
SVU	Society for Vascular Ultrasound
TAANA	The American Association of Nurse Attorneys
USPHS	United States Public Health Service
VA	Veterans Affairs
WHO	World Health Organization

Professional Designations for Health Care Providers*

Degrees, certifications, and memberships and other affiliations denoted by initials that precede or follow the names of health care providers often provide helpful information regarding their area of expertise and level of practice. The following list includes commonly used designations in English-speaking countries.

AIRC	Association of Insurance Regulation
AN	Associate Nurse
ANP	Adult Nurse Practitioner
APRN, BC	Advanced Practice Registered Nurse, Board Certified
ARNP	Advanced Registered Nurse Practitioner
ARRT	American Registry of Radiologic Technologists
ASCW	Academy of Certified Social Workers
BA	Bachelor of Arts
BB(ASCP)	Technologist in Blood Banking certified by the American Society of Clinical Pathologists
BDentSci	Bachelor of Dental Science
BDS	Bachelor of Dental Surgery
BDSc	Bachelor of Dental Science
BHS	Bachelor of Health Science
BHyg	Bachelor of Hygiene
BM	Bachelor of Medicine

*Modified from Miller-Keane Encyclopedia & Dictionary of Medicine, Nursing, & Allied Health, 7th ed., revised reprint. Philadelphia, Saunders, 2005.

BMed	Bachelor of Medicine
BMedBiol	Bachelor of Medical Biology
BMedSci	Bachelor of Medical Science
BMic	Bachelor of Microbiology
BMS	Bachelor of Medical Science
BMT	Bachelor of Medical Technology
BO	Bachelor of Osteopathy
BP	Bachelor of Pharmacy
BPH	Bachelor of Public Health
BPharm	Bachelor of Pharmacy
BPHEng	Bachelor of Public Health Engineering
BPHN	Bachelor of Public Health Nursing
BPsTh	Bachelor of Psychotherapy
BS	Bachelor of Science
BSM	Bachelor of Science in Medicine
BSN	Bachelor of Science in Nursing
BSPh	Bachelor of Science in Pharmacy
BSS	Bachelor of Sanitary Science
BVMS	Bachelor of Veterinary Medicine and Science
BVSc	Bachelor of Veterinary Science
CAC	Certified Alcohol Counselor
CALN	Clinical Administrative Liaison Nurse
CANP	Certified Adult Nurse Practitioner
C(ASCP)	Technologist in Chemistry certified by the American Society for Clinical Pathology
CB	Bachelor of Surgery
CCRN	Critical Care Registered Nurse
CCT	Certified Cardiographic Technician
CDA	Certified Dental Assistant
CDC	Certified Drug Counselor
CEN	Certificate for Emergency Nursing
CEO	Chief Executive Officer
CFNP	Certified Family Nurse Practitioner
ChB	Bachelor of Surgery

PROFESSIONAL DESIGNATIONS FOR HEALTH CARE PROVIDERS
(Continued)

ChD	Doctor of Surgery
CHES	Certified Health Education Specialist
ChM	Master of Surgery
CIC	Certified in Infection Control
CIH	Certificate in Industrial Health
CLA	Certified Laboratory Assistant
CLS	Clinical Laboratory Scientist
CLS(NCA)	Clinical Laboratory Scientist certified by the National Credentialing Agency for Medical Laboratory Personnel
CLT	Certified Laboratory Technician; Clinical Laboratory Technician
CLT(NCA)	Laboratory Technician certified by the National Credentialing Agency for Medical Laboratory Personnel
CM	Master of Surgery
CMA	Certified Medical Assistant
CMO	Chief Medical Officer
CMT	Chief Medical Transcriptionist
CNA	Certified Nursing Assistant
CNM	Certified Nurse-Midwife
CNMT	Certified Nuclear Medicine Technologist
CNOR	Certified Nurse, Operating Room
CNP	Community Nurse Practitioner
CNS	Clinical Nurse Specialist
CORN	Certified Operating Room Nurse
CORT	Certified Operating Room Technician
COTA	Certified Occupational Therapy Assistant
CPAN	Certified Peri-Anesthesia Nurse
CPH	Certified in Public Health
CPNP	Certified Pediatric Nurse Practitioner

CPTA	Certified Physical Therapy Assistant
CRNA	Certified Registered Nurse Anesthetist
CRNP	Certified Registered Nurse Practitioner
CRRN	Certified Registered Rehabilitation Nurse
CRRT	Certified Registered Respiratory Therapist
CRTT	Certified Respiratory Therapy Technician
CSN	Certified School Nurse
CT(ASCP)	Cytotechnologist certified by the American Society for Clinical Pathology
CURN	Certified Urological Registered Nurse
CVO	Chief Veterinary Officer
DA	Dental Assistant; Diploma in Anesthetics
DC	Doctor of Chiropractic
DCH	Diplomate in Child Health
DCh	Doctor of Surgery
DChO	Doctor of Ophthalmic Surgery
DCM	Doctor of Comparative Medicine
DCOG	Diplomate of the College of Obstetricians and Gynaecologists
DCP	Diplomate in Clinical Pathology; Diplomate in Clinical Psychology
DDH	Diplomate in Dental Health
DDM	Doctor of Dental Medicine; Diplomate in Dermatologic Medicine
DDO	Diplomate in Dental Orthopaedics
DDR	Diplomate in Dental Radiology
DDS	Doctor of Dental Surgery
DDSc	Doctor of Dental Science

DFHom	Diplomate in the Faculty of Homeopathy
DHg	Doctor of Hygiene
DHy	Doctor of Hygiene
DHyg	Doctor of Hygiene
Dipl	Diplomate
DipBact	Diplomate in Bacteriology
DipChem	Diplomate in Chemistry
DipClinPath	Diplomate in Clinical Pathology
DipMicrobiol	Diplomate in Microbiology
DipSocMed	Diplomate in Social Medicine
DLM(ASCP)	Diplomate in Laboratory Management of the American Society of Clinical Pathology
DMD	Doctor of Dental Medicine
DMT	Doctor of Medical Technology
DMV	Doctor of Veterinary Medicine
DN	Doctor of Nursing
DNE	Doctor of Nursing Education
DNS	Doctor of Nursing Science
DNSc	Doctor of Nursing Science
DO	Doctor of Ophthalmology; Doctor of Optometry; Doctor of Osteopathy
DON	Doctor of Nursing
DOS	Doctor of Ocular Science; Doctor of Optical Science
DP	Doctor of Pharmacy; Doctor of Podiatry
DPH	Doctor of Public Health; Doctor of Public Hygiene
DPhC	Doctor of Pharmaceutical Chemistry
DPHN	Doctor of Public Health Nursing
DPhys	Diplomate in Physiotherapy
DPM	Doctor of Physical Medicine; Doctor of Podiatric Medicine; Doctor of Preventive Medicine; Doctor of Psychiatric Medicine

Dr.	Doctor
DrHyg	Doctor of Hygiene
DrMed	Doctor of Medicine
DrPH	Doctor of Public Health; Doctor of Public Hygiene
DSc	Doctor of Science
DSE	Doctor of Sanitary Engineering
DSIM	Doctor of Science in Industrial Medicine
DSSc	Diplomate in Sanitary Science
DVM	Doctor of Veterinary Medicine
DVMS	Doctor of Veterinary Medicine and Surgery
DVR	Doctor of Veterinary Radiology
DVS	Doctor of Veterinary Science; Doctor of Veterinary Surgery
DVSc	Doctor of Veterinary Science
EdD	Doctor of Education
EMT	Emergency Medical Technician
EMT-P	Emergency Medical Technician–Paramedic
ET	Enterostomal Therapist
FAAN	Fellow of the American Academy of Nursing
FACA	Fellow of the American College of Anesthetists; Fellow of the American College of Angiology; Fellow of the American College of Apothecaries
FACAAI	Fellow of the American College of Allergy, Asthma and Immunology
FACC	Fellow of the American College of Cardiology
FACCP	Fellow of the American College of Chest Physicians
FACD	Fellow of the American College of Dentists
FACFP	Fellow of the American College of Family Physicians

FACG	Fellow of the American College of Gastroenterology
FACHA	Fellow of the American College of Health Administrators
FACOG	Fellow of the American College of Obstetricians and Gynecologists
FACP	Fellow of the American College of Physicians
FACPM	Fellow of the American College of Preventive Medicine
FACS	Fellow of the American College of Surgeons
FACSM	Fellow of the American College of Sports Medicine
FAMA	Fellow of the American Medical Association
FAOTA	Fellow of the American Occupational Therapy Association
FAPA	Fellow of the American Psychiatric Association
FAPHA	Fellow of the American Public Health Association
FBPsS	Fellow of the British Psychological Society
FCAP	Fellow of the College of American Pathologists
FCO	Fellow of the College of Osteopathy
FCPS	Fellow of the College of Physicians and Surgeons
FCSP	Fellow of the Chartered Society of Physiotherapy
FCST	Fellow of the College of Speech Therapists
FDS	Fellow in Dental Surgery

FFA	Fellow of the Faculty of Anesthetists
FFCM	Fellow of the Faculty of Community Medicine
FFD	Fellow of the Faculty of Dentistry
FFOM	Fellow of the Faculty of Occupational Medicine
FFR	Fellow of the Faculty of Radiologists
FIB	Fellow of the Institute of Biology
FICD	Fellow of the Institute of Canadian Dentists; Fellow of the International College of Dentists
FIMLT	Fellow of Institute of Medical Laboratory Technology
FNP	Family Nurse Practitioner
GNP	Gerontological Nurse Practitioner
H(ASCP)	Technologist in Hematology certified by the American Society for Clinical Pathology
HT(ASCP)	Histologic Technician certified by the American Society for Clinical Pathology
HTL(ASCP)	Histotechnologist certified by the American Society for Clinical Pathology
I(ASCP)	Technologist in Immunology certified by the American Society for Clinical Pathology
LCSW	Licensed Clinical Social Worker
LMCC	Licentiate of the Medical Council of Canada
LMRCP	Licentiate in Midwifery of the Royal College of Physicians
LOT	Licensed Occupational Therapist
LPN	Licensed Practical Nurse
LPT	Licensed Physical Therapist
LVN	Licensed Vocational Nurse

PROFESSIONAL DESIGNATIONS FOR HEALTH CARE PROVIDERS
(Continued)

MA	Master of Arts
M(ASCP)	Technologist in Microbiology certified by the American Society for Clinical Pathology
MB	Bachelor of Medicine
MC	Master of Surgery
MCIS	Master of Computer and Information Science; Master of Computer Information Systems
MCPS	Member of the College of Physicians and Surgeons
MD	Doctor of Medicine
MDentSc	Master of Dental Science
MDS	Master of Dental Surgery
MHC	Mental Health Counselor
MLT	Medical Laboratory Technician
MLT(ASCP)	Medical Laboratory Technician certified by the American Society for Clinical Pathology
MMID	Master of Midwifery
MMS	Master of Medical Science
MPH	Master of Public Health
MPharm	Master of Pharmacy
MRad	Master of Radiology
MRL	Medical Records Librarian
MS	Master of Science; Master of Surgery
MSB	Master of Science in Bacteriology
MSc	Master of Science
MScD	Master of Dental Science
MScN	Master of Science in Nursing
MSN	Master of Science in Nursing
MSPH	Master of Science in Public Health
MSPhar	Master of Science in Pharmacy
MSSc	Master of Sanitary Science
MSW	Master of Social Work; Medical Social Worker
MT	Medical Technologist

PROFESSIONAL DESIGNATIONS FOR HEALTH CARE PROVIDERS
(Continued)

MT(ASCP)	Medical Technologist certified by the American Society for Clinical Pathology
MVD	Doctor of Veterinary Medicine
NA	Nursing Aide
ND	Doctor of Nursing
NHA	Nursing Home Administrator
NM(ASCP)	Technologist in Nuclear Medicine certified by the American Society for Clinical Pathology
NMT	Nuclear Medicine Technologist
NNP	Neonatal Nurse Practitioner
NP	Nurse Practitioner
OD	Doctor of Optometry
ONC	Orthopedic Nursing Certificate
ORT	Operating Room Technician
OT	Occupational Therapist
OTL	Occupational Therapist, Licensed
OTR	Occupational Therapist, Registered
OTReg	Occupational Therapist, Registered
PA	Physician Assistant
PA-C	Physician Assistant–Certified
PBT(ASCP)	Phlebotomy Technician certified by the American Society for Clinical Pathology
PCP	Primary Care Physician
PD	Doctor of Pharmacy
PharmD	Doctor of Pharmacy
PhD	Doctor of Philosophy; Doctor of Pharmacy
PHN	Public Health Nurse
PNP	Pediatric Nurse Practitioner
PT	Physical Therapist
PTA	Physical Therapy Assistant
RD	Registered Dietician
RDA	Registered Dental Assistant
RDMS	Registered Diagnostic Medical Sonographer

REEGT	Registered Electroencephalographic Technologist
Reg	Registered
RHIA	Registered Health Information Administrator
RHIT	Registered Health Information Technician
RMA	Registered Medical Assistant
RN	Registered Nurse
RNA	Registered Nurse Anesthetist
RN, BC	Registered Nurse, Board Certified
RN, C	Registered Nurse, Certified
RN, CNA	Registered Nurse, Certified in Nursing Administration
RN, CNAA	Registered Nurse, Certified in Nursing Administration, Advanced
RN, CNA, BC	Registered Nurse, Certified in Nursing Administration, Board Certified
RN, CS	Registered Nurse, Certified Specialist
RPh	Registered Pharmacist
RPT	Registered Physical Therapist
RPTA	Registered Physical Therapist Assistant
RRL	Registered Record Librarian
RRT	Registered Respiratory Therapist
RT	Radiologic Technologist; Respiratory Therapist
RT(N)	Nuclear Medicine Technologist
RT(R)	Technologist in Diagnostic Radiology
RTR	Registered Recreational Therapist
RT(T)	Radiation Therapy Technologist
SBB(ASCP)	Specialist in Blood Banking certified by the American Society for Clinical Pathology

PROFESSIONAL DESIGNATIONS FOR HEALTH CARE PROVIDERS
(Continued)

ScD	Doctor of Science
SCT(ASCP)	Specialist in Cytotechnology certified by the American Society for Clinical Pathology
SLP	Speech-Language Pathologist
SNP	School Nurse Practitioner
ST	Speech Therapist; Surgical Technologist
SW	Social Worker

Surgical Terminology and Technology*

The following terms are commonly used in surgery and anesthesia. They include terms related to surgical and anesthetic instrumentation and procedures.

TERM	DEFINITION
ablation	Removal by erosion or vaporization, usually due to intense heat.
abscess	Localized area of pus in the body.
absorbable suture	Any suture that can be digested by body tissue.
ampule	Small glass container that holds medication that has been sterilized.
analgesia	Absence of pain.
anastomosis	Surgical formation of a passageway between two spaces, hollow organs, or lumens.
anesthetic	Agent that produces analgesia.
appose	To bring two structures together.
approximate	To bring body parts or tissues together by suturing or other means.
armboard	Detachable extension on the operating table that supports the patient's arm.

*Modified from Fuller JR: Surgical Technology: Principles and Practice, 5th ed. Philadelphia, Saunders, 2010.

SURGICAL TERMINOLOGY AND
TECHNOLOGY (Continued)

TERM	DEFINITION
aspirate	To withdraw fluids or gases by means of suction, as when removing fluid from the body with a syringe; also refers to the material thus obtained.
atraumatic	Referring to a suture-needle combination in which the suture is swaged into the end of the needle shaft, rather than threaded through a needle eye, with its typical bulge; the needle thus passes more readily through tissue.
autoclave	Steam sterilizer.
autotransfusion	Transfusion using the patient's own blood.
Bankart procedure	Operation on the shoulder girdle to treat recurrent shoulder dislocation.
bifurcated	Y-shaped; divided into two branches.
biopsy	Removal of a small piece of tissue from a living body for microscopic examination.
bipolar	Refers to a type of electrosurgical unit in which the electrical current is localized at the tip of the electrocautery probe and does not pass through the patient.
bipolar coagulation	Electrosurgery that utilizes forceps rather than an electrosurgical pencil.
bleeder	Severed blood vessel.

SURGICAL TERMINOLOGY AND TECHNOLOGY (Continued)

TERM	DEFINITION
blunt dissection	Separation of tissues or tissue planes with an instrument that has no cutting ability.
bolster	Tubing through which retention sutures are threaded to prevent them from cutting into the patient's skin.
bone wax	Medical-grade beeswax used on bone tissue to control bleeding.
Bovie cleaner	Small, rough-surfaced pad used to clean the electrocautery tip during surgery.
box lock	Ratchet closure mechanism of many surgical instruments.
Brown and Sharpe (B&S) wire gauge	Sizing standard used to measure steel sutures.
bur	Round instrument with sharp cutting edges used for drilling holes in bone.
caliper	Orthopedic device for measuring the width of a ball joint head in preparation for a prosthetic implant.
capillary action	Physical mechanism by which liquids are absorbed along the length of a suture.
case assignments	Written schedule of each surgical team member's assigned cases for the day.
caudal	Toward the feet.

SURGICAL TERMINOLOGY AND
TECHNOLOGY (Continued)

TERM	DEFINITION
caudal anesthetic	Anesthetic agent introduced into the caudal canal to induce a type of epidural anesthesia.
chromic salts	Chemicals used to treat surgical gut suture so that it resists digestion by body tissues.
circulator	Surgical team member who does not perform a surgical hand scrub or don sterile attire and thus does not work within the sterile field.
clamp	Instrument designed to hold tissue, objects (such as surgical needles), or fabric (such as a towel).
cleaning	Process that removes organic or inorganic debris.
closed anesthesia system	In general anesthesia, the recirculation of anesthetic gases through the gas machine and back to the patient, which prevents exposure of personnel to the gases.
closed gloving	Method of donning sterile gloves when a surgical gown is worn.
closed reduction	Process in which bone fragments are reduced manually, without surgical intervention.
coagulation	Clotting of blood.
communicate	To connect; used to describe the relationship between two structures or organs that connect.

SURGICAL TERMINOLOGY AND TECHNOLOGY (Continued)

TERM	DEFINITION
curette	Spoon-shaped instrument used to scrape tissue from a surface.
cutting instrument	Any instrument with a sharp edge.
dead space	Area lying between tissue layers or opposing them that the surgeon has not approximated; dead space within a wound can lead to infection.
débridement	Process of removing dead skin, debris, or foreign bodies from a wound.
defibrillator	Piece of equipment used to generate electrical impulses to the heart during cardiac arrest in an attempt to restart the heartbeat.
deflect	To peel or retract back and away but not detach.
dehiscence	Splitting apart of a surgical wound after surgery.
dermabrasion	Physical sanding of the skin to remove pockmarks and other scars.
desiccation	Drying up of a substance.
dilators	Graduated, rodlike instruments used to enlarge the diameter of a channel or duct.
dissector	Tiny sponge mounted on a clamp and used to perform blunt dissection.
divide	To cut or sever.

SURGICAL TERMINOLOGY AND
TECHNOLOGY (Continued)

TERM	DEFINITION
dorsal recumbent	Position of the patient lying on his or her back; synonymous with *supine*.
drill bit	In orthopedics, an instrument used in a drill to create a hole in bone to accommodate a screw.
emergence	Arousal from general anesthesia after cessation of the anesthetic agent.
endotracheal tube	Tube that is inserted into the patient's trachea for the administration of anesthetic gas.
endotracheal tube fire	Fire that occurs within the patient's endotracheal tube during laser surgery, which causes immediate and severe trauma to the lungs.
epidural anesthetic	Type of anesthetic agent that is introduced into the epidural space of the spine.
Esmarch bandage	Rolled rubber bandage that is wrapped around the limb to force blood away from the surgical site before the application of a tourniquet.
ethylene oxide gas	Highly flammable, toxic gas that is capable of sterilizing an object
evisceration	In surgery, the splitting open of an abdominal surgical wound and subsequent spillage of its contents.
excise	To remove by cutting out.

SURGICAL TERMINOLOGY AND TECHNOLOGY (Continued)

TERM	DEFINITION
excitement	Second stage of general anesthesia in which the patient is sensitive to external stimuli.
exposure	Anatomic area that the surgeon can see and thus operate on.
extractor	In orthopedics, an instrument used to remove a metal implant from bone.
fiberoptic	Refers to a flexible material that carries light along its length, composed of fibers of glass or plastic that are bundled together to form the cables used for endoscopic examination.
first intention	Process by which a clean surgical wound heals directly, without granulation.
fistula	Abnormal passageway from a normal cavity to the outside of the body or another cavity.
fixation	In orthopedics, to hold bone fragments in place following a fracture; in *external* fixation, the fragments are held in alignment by an external device, such as a plaster cast; in *internal* fixation, fragments are held in alignment with an appliance such as a rod, nail, or screw.
flaking	Tendency of some suture materials to release tiny particles of the suture in the wound.

SURGICAL TERMINOLOGY AND
TECHNOLOGY (Continued)

TERM	DEFINITION
flash autoclave	Autoclave used in surgery to sterilize equipment quickly by steam under pressure.
footboard	Section of the operating table at the foot end that can be removed or angled up or down.
four-by-four (4 × 4)	Type of surgical sponge, 4 inches square, consisting of loosely woven gauze.
Fowler position	Sitting position.
fracture	Breaking of a part of the body, especially bone; different types of fractures include (1) comminuted—the bone is splintered into many small fragments; (2) compound—the fracture penetrates adjacent soft tissue and skin (also called an open fracture); (3) greenstick—the fracture extends only partially through the bone; incomplete; (4) impacted—a portion of the bone is traumatically driven into another bone or fragment; (5) pathologic—caused by disease rather than injury; (6) spiral—forms a spiral pattern; bone has been twisted apart; (7) transverse—the fracture line lies perpendicular to the long axis of the bone.

SURGICAL TERMINOLOGY AND TECHNOLOGY (Continued)

TERM	DEFINITION
free tie	Term used by the surgeon in requesting a length of suture for ligation.
French-eye	Delicate needle whose eye contains a spring.
friable	Refers to any tissue that is easily torn.
frozen section	Fine slice of frozen biopsy tissue; submitted for microscopic examination for the presence of disease.
full length	Refers to the length of a suture strand; full length is 54 or 60 inches.
gas	Matter in its least dense state; air at room temperature is a gas.
gauge	In orthopedics, an instrument used to measure the depth of a hole made by a drill bit.
Gelfoam	Medical-grade gelatin foam that is used to control capillary bleeding.
general anesthetic	Type of anesthetic agent that causes unconsciousness.
glutaraldehyde	Chemical capable of rendering objects sterile.
gouge	In orthopedic surgery, an instrument used to create a grooved surface on bone.
gravity displacement sterilizer	Type of sterilizer that removes air by gravity.
grounding cable	During electrosurgery, the cable connecting the control unit to the inactive electrode.

SURGICAL TERMINOLOGY AND
TECHNOLOGY (Continued)

TERM	DEFINITION
grounding pad	Gel-covered pad that grounds the patient during electrosurgery; inactive electrode.
gurney	Type of wheeled stretcher used for patient transport to or within a clinical facility.
headboard	Removable section of the operating table at the head end that can be angled up or down.
hemostasis	The control of hemorrhage during surgery.
hemostat	Instrument used to clamp a blood vessel.
hemostatic agent	Drug that promotes blood coagulation.
high-vacuum sterilizer	Type of steam sterilizer that removes air in the chamber by vacuum.
impactor	In orthopedics, an instrument used to drive an implant into bone; also may be called a *driver*.
incise	To cut or sever with a cutting instrument.
induction	First stage of general anesthesia during which the patient's physiologic status is unstable.
inflammation	Localized, protective reaction of tissue to injury or disease.
infusion pump	Containment and monitoring equipment used when the patient receives intravenous solutions, including anesthetics.

SURGICAL TERMINOLOGY AND TECHNOLOGY (Continued)

TERM	DEFINITION
intentional hypotension	During surgery, the intentional lowering of a patient's blood pressure to control hemorrhage.
intentional hypothermia	During surgery, the intentional lowering of a patient's core temperature to control hemorrhage.
Javid shunt	Commercially prepared length of plastic tubing used to bypass the carotid artery temporarily during carotid endarterectomy.
jaws	Working end of a clasping- or gripping-type surgical instrument.
Kerlix bandage	Rolled bandage made of soft, woven material.
Kraske position	Operative position used for procedures on the perianal area; the patient lies in prone position, with the table broken at its midsection so that the head and feet are lower than the midsection; also called *jackknife position* or *knee-chest position.*
laminectomy position	Operative position used for spinal surgery; a form of the prone position.
laparotomy tape	Largest surgical sponge available, used during major surgery; also called a *lap tape.*

SURGICAL TERMINOLOGY AND
TECHNOLOGY (Continued)

TERM	DEFINITION
laser	Acronym for light amplification by stimulated emission of radiation; a device that generates a beam of extremely bright light of a single color.
lateral	Refers to a side; for example, the little toe lies on the lateral aspect of the foot.
lavage	Irrigation of body cavities; during malignant hyperthermia, cold saline lavage is used to lower the patient's temperature.
ligate	To tie a length of suture around a vessel or duct and secure it with knots.
ligation clips	Small V-shaped clips that are applied around blood vessels or ducts in place of a ligature; sometimes referred to as *silver clips*.
local anesthetic	Type of anesthetic agent that causes loss of sensation or feeling in a localized area.
local infiltration	Procedure in which the anesthetic is injected directly into the operative tissue.
lumen	Hollow tube.
malignant hyperthermia	Anesthetic-related phenomenon that causes the patient's temperature to rise suddenly and become critically high; emergency procedures are initiated during this crisis.

SURGICAL TERMINOLOGY AND TECHNOLOGY (Continued)

TERM	DEFINITION
memory	Suture's ability to "remember" its manufactured configuration after removal from packaging (e.g., coiled or twisted).
microfibrillar collagen hemostat	Substance derived from collagen and used as a hemostatic agent.
monitored anesthesia care	Procedure in which the patient receives an intravenous sedative anesthetic, which may be given in conjunction with a local anesthetic or by itself.
monofilament suture	Suture composed of a single, nonfibrous strand of material.
monopolar	Refers to a type of electrosurgical unit in which the electrical current passes through the patient and back to the control unit.
multifilament suture	Suture composed of many fine strands of fiber that are twisted or braided together.
nail	Orthopedic device used to fasten together pieces of bone; examples are Neufeld nail, Jewett nail, Ken sliding nail, and Smith-Petersen nail.
necrotic	Referring to dead tissue.
nerve block	Anesthesia of a large single nerve or nerves.
neuromuscular blocking agent	Pharmaceutical agent that causes paralysis and is used for this purpose during general anesthesia.

SURGICAL TERMINOLOGY AND TECHNOLOGY (Continued)

TERM	DEFINITION
nonabsorbable suture	Suture that is never digested by tissue but becomes encapsulated by it.
open gloving	Method of donning sterile surgical gloves when a gown is not worn.
open reduction	Realignment of bone fragments with surgical instruments.
orthopedic cutdown instruments	Instruments used to gain access to fractures or to operate on soft tissue injuries; examples are scalpel handles, tissue forceps, Metzenbaum scissors, Mayo scissors, needle holders, mosquito clamps, Allis clamps, Kelly clamps, Kocher clamps, and Mayo clamps.
orthopedic cutting instruments	Instruments used to cut bone; examples are rasps (to smooth the surface of a bone or remove the medullary cavity so a stemmed prosthesis can be inserted), reamers (used to form hollow area in the bone), knives (used to cut away heavy connective tissue such as cartilage), elevators (used to lift the periosteum from the surface of the bone or to perform fine dissection during tendon and ligament repair), rongeurs (used to cut bone), saws (power-driven and used to cut through fine bone), osteotomes (used to create

SURGICAL TERMINOLOGY AND TECHNOLOGY (Continued)

TERM	DEFINITION
	slivers of bone used in a graft), curettes (used to spoon out bits of bone from a curved area), gouges (used to create a grooved surface on the bone), and drills (used in conjunction with a drill bit to drill a hole).
orthopedic internal fixation devices	Surgical steel or alloy appliances used to stabilize a fracture during healing; examples are pins and bolts, nails, plates, staples, and screws.
orthopedic measuring devices	Instruments used in implant procedures; examples are calipers (used to measure the width of a ball joint head in preparation for a prosthetic implant) and depth gauges (used to measure the depth of the hole made by a drill to determine what length of screw is needed).
osteotome	Chisel-like instrument used with a mallet to cut bone.
oxidized cellulose	Medical-grade cellulose manufactured into mesh squares and used as a hemostatic agent.
PACU	Acronym for **p**ost**a**nesthesia **c**are **u**nit.
patty	Type of sponge used during neurosurgery.
peracetic acid	Chemical capable of rendering objects sterile.

SURGICAL TERMINOLOGY AND TECHNOLOGY (Continued)

TERM	DEFINITION
pin	Device used in orthopedics to fasten together pieces of bone; pins are inserted with a drill or driver; examples are Steinmann pin and Knowles pin; also used as a verb, meaning to secure and immobilize fragments of bone.
plate	Orthopedic flat internal fixation device held in place with screws; examples are adjustable McLaughlin plate, Moe intertrochanteric plate, and Bagby compression plate.
points	Tips of a surgical instrument.
precut	Lengths of suture material that are cut to a standard length by the manufacturer.
probe	Instrument placed within a lumen to determine its length and direction.
prosthesis	Any artificial organ or body part.
pursestring	Technique of suturing; a continuous strand is passed in and out around the circumference of a hollow structure and then is pulled tight like a drawstring.
ratchets	Interlocking clasps that hold a finger ring instrument closed.

SURGICAL TERMINOLOGY AND TECHNOLOGY (Continued)

TERM	DEFINITION
reamer	Instrument used in orthopedic surgery to create a hollow area in bone.
reduce	In orthopedics, to bring two bone fragments in alignment after a fracture.
reel	Continuous strand of suture mounted on a spool; used for ligation of many blood vessels in rapid succession.
relaxation	During general anesthesia, the operative phase.
resect	To cut out and remove a section of tissue.
retention suture	Heavy, nonabsorbable suture placed behind the skin sutures and underneath all tissue layers to give added strength to the closure.
retract	To pull tissues back or away to expose a structure or other tissue.
reverse Trendelenburg position	Operative position in which the patient lies supine and the operating table is tilted so that the head is higher than the feet.
running suture	Method of suturing that uses one continuous suture that is passed over and under the tissue edges.
self-tapping shank	In orthopedics, a screw that creates its own hole in bone as it is being inserted.
shank	Area of a surgical instrument between the box lock and the finger ring.

SURGICAL TERMINOLOGY AND
TECHNOLOGY (Continued)

TERM	DEFINITION
sharp dissection	Use of a scalpel or other sharp instrument for the separation of tissues.
shelf life	Amount of time a wrapped object will remain sterile after it has been subjected to a sterilization process.
Sims position	Position in which the patient lies on the side with the upper leg drawn up; also called *lateral position*.
sizer	Dummy or model of a prosthesis used during an operation to determine the correct size of prosthesis needed.
specimen	Any tissue, foreign body, prosthesis, or fluid that is removed from the patient.
speculum	Instrument used for exposure of a body cavity, such as the nasal passages.
sponge stick	Folded four-by-four mounted on a sponge clamp.
steam sterilizer	Sterilizer that exposes objects to high-pressure steam.
sterile	Completely free of living microorganisms.
sterile field	Area that encompasses draped equipment, scrubbed personnel, and the draped patient.
stick tie	Name given to suture ligature—a suture-needle combination that is passed through a vessel or duct before ligation to prevent it from slipping off the edge of the structure.

SURGICAL TERMINOLOGY AND TECHNOLOGY (Continued)

TERM	DEFINITION
surgeon's preference card	File card that contains information pertaining to suture materials, equipment, or special instruments used by a particular surgeon.
surgical drape	Sterile cloth or nonwoven material placed around the surgical site to create a sterile field.
surgical scrub	Precise method by which all team members who will be working in sterile attire scrub their hands and arms before performing an operation.
surgically clean	As clean as possible without being sterile.
suture	Material used to bring tissues together by sewing; also can refer to a suture-needle combination.
suture ligature	Needle-suture combination used to tie a bleeding vessel and attach it to nearby tissue simultaneously, thus preventing the tie from slipping off the end of the vessel.
table breaks	Hinged sections of the operating table that can be folded up or down to create different postures.
tenaculum	Instrument used to grasp tissue.

SURGICAL TERMINOLOGY AND
TECHNOLOGY (Continued)

TERM	DEFINITION
tensile strength	Amount of stress a suture will withstand before breaking.
terminal disinfection	Process in which an area or object is rendered disinfected after contamination has occurred.
tie-on passer	Strand of suture material whose end is secured to the end of a long clamp; used to ligate deep vessels when exposure is limited.
topical anesthetic	Drug used on the surface of tissue, such as the eye.
topical thrombin	Drug used in conjunction with gelatin sponges to halt capillary bleeding.
torsion	Twisting of an organ or structure upon itself, which often causes diminished blood supply to the affected area.
tourniquet	Device that prevents the flow of blood to the surgical wound.
transect	To cut across an organ or section of tissue.
Trendelenburg position	Operative position in which the patient lies in supine position with the operating table tilted so that the head is lower than the feet.
trocar	Spear-shaped instrument or needle.

SURGICAL TERMINOLOGY AND TECHNOLOGY (Continued)

TERM	DEFINITION
ultrasonic cleaner	Equipment that cleans instruments through cavitation.
washer-sterilizer	Equipment that washes and sterilizes instruments after an operative procedure.
Webril	Soft, rolled cotton material used to pad a limb before the application of a plaster cast.

Complementary and Alternative Medicine Terms*

Following is a listing of common complementary and alternative medicine (CAM) terms. A comprehensive listing of CAM terms, as well as more information on some of the terms listed here, can be found in *Mosby's Dictionary of Complementary and Alternative Medicine*.

Note: The practice of any complementary or alternative medicine techniques and the use of any herbal remedies should be approached with caution and care, or under the supervision of a CAM professional or your physician.

acupoints	Particular locations on the body that allow the practitioner to balance the client's qi (life force) to effect therapeutic changes using acupuncture or acupressure.
acupressure	Technique used to release blocked qi (life force) by applying finger pressure to points on meridians.
acupuncture	Practice in Chinese medicine (developed more than 2000 years ago) in which the skin, at various points along meridians, is punctured with needles to remove energy blockages and to stimulate the flow of qi (life force).

---

*Excerpts from Jonas WB: Mosby's Dictionary of Complementary and Alternative Medicine. St. Louis, Mosby, 2005; and http://nccam.nih.gov/health/bytreatment.htm#s1, on the website of National Center for Complementary and Alternative Medicine of the National Institutes of Health.

Complementary and Alternative Medicine Terms (Continued)

aloe	This plant's leaves are used to treat minor burns, wounds, skin and GI disorders, menstrual cramps, premenstrual syndrome, and other ailments.
antioxidants	Substances that may protect cells from damage caused by unstable molecules known as free radicals. Such damage may lead to cancer, aging, and other conditions. Examples of antioxidants are beta-carotene and vitamins C, E, and A.
apiotherapy	Use of products produced by honeybees, including pollen and venom, for therapeutic and pharmacologic purposes.
applied kinesiology	Physical therapy model that draws on various therapeutic schools of thought. The aim of this therapy is the recovery of muscles that are functionally inhibited with respect to normal range of motion and strength (possibly as a result of disturbances in the nervous or neuromuscular system).
aromatherapy	Use of essential oils (extracts and essences) from flowers, herbs, and trees applied topically or inhaled to promote and maintain overall health.

Complementary and Alternative Medicine Terms (Continued)

ayurvedic medicine	Also known as *ayurveda*—meaning the science (*veda*) of life (*ayu*). It is an ancient Indian health system that works to reestablish the balance between the body and the mind (uses diet, herbal remedies, meditation, massage, and other modalities).
bilberry	Used to treat myopia, retinal problems, inflammation of the mouth and pharynx, GI disorders, varicose veins, and other ailments.
biofeedback	Process in which equipment sensors provide measurements of body functions (such as heart rate or neural activity), and those signals are displayed to the patient, to permit conscious control of the measured function.
black cohosh	Its roots are used to treat menopause, menstrual cramps, diarrhea, and other ailments.
chamomile	This plant's dried buds are used to treat inflammatory disease of the GI and upper respiratory tracts and inflammation of the skin and mucous membranes; to promote healing of wounds, rashes, and ulcers (applied topically); and to relieve motion sickness, GI spasms, restlessness, nervousness or insomnia, and other ailments.

Complementary and Alternative Medicine Terms (Continued)

chelation therapy
Medical treatment in which heavy metals are flushed from the bloodstream by means of a chelator that binds metal ions; used in cases of mercury or lead poisoning.

chi
In Tibetan medicine, awareness, one of the three functions of the mind, providing the direction for actions.

chiropractic therapy
Health discipline focusing on the relationship between body structure (primarily of the spine) and function. Chiropractors use manipulative therapy to treat the client's back, neck, and limbs.

chondroitin
Naturally occurring substance responsible for cartilage repair and taken as a dietary supplement. Used with glucosamine for knee osteoarthritis.

circadian rhythm
The biologic patterns (of a specific person) within a 24-hour cycle, over the course of a day.

coenzyme Q10
Compound, made naturally in the body, that is used for cell growth and to protect cells from damage. The dietary supplement is used to help the immune system work better, especially during the treatment of cancer and heart failure.

Complementary and Alternative Medicine Terms (Continued)

complementary and alternative medicine (CAM)	Group of diverse medical and health care systems, practices, and products that at present are not considered part of conventional or mainstream medicine. Complementary medicine is used **together with** conventional medicine (e.g., aromatherapy to lessen patient discomfort after surgery). Alternative medicine is used **in place of** conventional medicine (e.g., the patient may choose to follow a special diet to address ADHD symptoms, rather than using drug therapy).
dehydroepiandrosterone (DHEA)	Hormone precursor that exists naturally in yams. Used to slow the effects of aging, to support or improve memory, and to treat erectile dysfunction, depression, osteoporosis, and atherosclerosis.
echinacea	This plant's roots, flowers, and leaves are used to treat upper respiratory and urinary tract infections, allergic rhinitis, and other ailments, and to promote wound healing.

**Complementary and Alternative
Medicine Terms** (Continued)

electromagnetic fields (EMFs)	Invisible lines of force that surround all electrical devices. Bioelectromagnetic-based therapies involve unconventional use of electromagnets, such as pulsed fields and magnetic currents, to treat chronic disease or to manage pain, especially migraine headaches.
ergonomics	Applied study of psychology, anatomy, and physiology relating to people and work environments.
folate	Water-soluble B vitamin that occurs naturally in food. Folic acid is the synthetic form of folate that is found in supplements and added to fortified foods. Folate helps produce and maintain new cells. This is especially important during periods of rapid cell division and growth, such as infancy and pregnancy.
garlic	This plant's bulbs are used to manage and treat hypercholesterolemia (elevated cholesterol levels), atherosclerosis, hypertension, upper respiratory tract infections, and other conditions.
ginger	This plant's roots are used to manage and treat nausea and vomiting, motion sickness, and other conditions.

Complementary and Alternative Medicine Terms (Continued)

ginkgo (*Ginkgo biloba*)
This plant's leaves are used to manage and treat Alzheimer disease, dementia, depression, asthma, retinal disease, heart disease, peripheral arterial occlusive disease, varicose veins, premenstrual syndrome, tinnitus, and other conditions.

ginseng
This plant's roots are used to manage and treat fatigue, stress, mild depression, decreased libido, and other conditions and ailments.

glucosamine
Amino sugar that the body produces and distributes in cartilage and other connective tissue. Glucosamine is used alone and in conjunction with chondroitin sulfate to treat knee osteoarthritis.

guided imagery
Directed relaxation and visualization, as well as exercises in self-relaxation and other beneficial practices, to support changes in health.

herbalism
Study and practice of using plants to treat illnesses and promote health; also called *phytotherapy*.

homeopathy
System of treating disease based on the administration of minute doses of a drug that in massive amounts produces symptoms in healthy persons similar to those of the disease itself.

Complementary and Alternative Medicine Terms (Continued)

hydrotherapy	Therapeutic modality that uses water, such as whirlpools or sitz baths.
integrative medicine	Combines mainstream medical therapies and CAM therapies for which there is some evidence for safety and effectiveness.
kava	This plant's rhizomes and roots are used to treat anxiety, restlessness, fibromyalgia, tension headaches, insomnia, alcohol dependence, and other ailments.
kinesiology	Study of the body's structure and processes as they relate to movement.
lymphatic drainage	Specific type of massage that supports and assists circulation in the lymphatic system.
macrobiotic diet	Designed to bring yin/yang energies into balance, the macrobiotic diet, developed by Michio Kushi, is part of a larger lifestyle/philosophy and whole-body regimen.
manipulation	In massage therapy, osteopathic medicine, chiropractic, and traditional Chinese medicine, the use of various manual techniques to adjust the joints and spinal column, improve the range of motion of the joints, relax and stretch connective tissue and muscles, and promote overall relaxation.

Complementary and Alternative Medicine Terms (Continued)

massage therapy
Application of diverse manual techniques of touch and stroking to muscles and soft tissue to achieve relaxation and to improve sense of well-being.

meditation
Directing one's attention toward a symbol, sound, thought, or breath to alter the state of consciousness, to attain a state of relaxation and stress relief; used for spiritual growth, healing, deepening concentration, and unlocking creativity.

melatonin
Hormone secreted from the pineal gland and thought to regulate circadian rhythms; also used in supplement form as a sleep aid.

meridians
In acupuncture, a system of pathways or channels running through the body that connect vital organs and carry qi.

milk thistle
This plant's seeds are used to make a tea to treat liver and gallbladder disease, hepatitis, and dyspepsia, and to support the liver during transplantation recovery.

Complementary and Alternative Medicine Terms (Continued)

mistletoe	Leafy shoots and berries of mistletoe are used to make extracts that can be taken by mouth. Mistletoe has been used for centuries to treat seizures, headaches, and other conditions. Clinical trials are ongoing for possible effects on cancer treatment.
naturopathy	Therapeutic system that relies on using natural agents such as light, natural foods, warmth, massage, and fresh air. Naturopaths believe in the power of the body's natural processes to heal illnesses.
omega-3 fatty acids	Group of polyunsaturated fatty acids that come from food sources such as fish, fish oil, some vegetable oils (primarily canola and soybean), walnuts, wheat germ, and certain dietary supplements. Clinical trials are ongoing to test the effects of omega-3 fatty acids on various conditions and for enhancement of general well-being.
osteopathy	Form of medicine that uses joint manipulation, physical therapy, and postural reeducation to restore the structural balance of the musculoskeletal system.

Complementary and Alternative Medicine Terms (Continued)

qi	Body's life force. In Chinese philosophy, qi is the force that flows through channels in the body and enlivens all living beings; an imbalance in qi is believed to cause illness.
qi gong	Cultivation of qi. *Qi gong* (chee-GUNG) is the general term for all Chinese techniques of breathing, visualization, and movement, the purpose of which is the promotion of balanced qi flow (vital energy) for enhanced immune function and blood flow.
reflexology	Natural healing system based on the principle that reflexes in the hands and feet correspond to various organs and body systems; stimulating such reflexes by applying pressure on hands and feet improves circulation, thereby optimizing body functions.
Reiki	System of spiritual healing/energy medicine developed by Japanese physician Dr. Mikao Usui. Reiki (RAY-Kee) is a Japanese word representing universal life energy. It is based on the belief that when spiritual energy is channeled through a Reiki practitioner, the patient's spirit is healed, which then heals the physical body.

**Complementary and Alternative
Medicine Terms** (Continued)

Rolfing	Ten-session manual therapy developed to optimize the body's movement and alignment and coordination with the forces of gravity, for relief of muscular and emotional tension.
selenium	Trace mineral that is essential to good health but required only in small amounts. Selenium is incorporated into proteins to make selenoproteins, which are important antioxidant enzymes. The antioxidant effects of selenoproteins help prevent cellular damage from free radicals. Free radicals are natural byproducts of oxygen metabolism that may contribute to the development of chronic diseases such as cancer and heart disease. Clinical trials are ongoing to test the effects of selenium in the treatment and prevention of cancer.
shiatsu	Type of massage developed in Japan; it consists of the application of pressure to specific points on the human body with the palms and thumbs.

Complementary and Alternative Medicine Terms (Continued)

soy
Soybeans ingested in various forms may support healthy body tissues by neutralizing free radicals. Soy may offer a diversity of antioxidant mechanisms.

St. John's wort
This plant's flowers may be used to treat mild to moderate depression, anxiety, sleep disorders, and other ailments.

tai chi
In traditional Chinese medicine, a family of health-promoting exercises that provide benefits for the body, mind, and soul by maintaining balance between the yin and yang components; these exercises comprise flowing movements that imitate the motions and forms of animals, all of which share fundamental elements rooted in qi gong.

valerian
This plant's rhizomes and roots are used to treat sleeping disorders, nervousness, anxiety, restlessness, irritable bowel syndrome, and other ailments.

yin and yang
Governing theory behind traditional Chinese medicine: the idea that life is filled with opposite yet complementary characteristics and qualities on the spiritual and physical levels and on the macro and micro levels. The concept is that each entity can be

Complementary and Alternative Medicine Terms (Continued)

essentially itself and its opposite; additionally, yang's "seed" is believed to be contained within yin; a balance of yin and yang is considered essential for good health, whereas an imbalance can manifest as disease.

yoga
Family of mind-body disciplines that share the goals of the integrated body and mind or the union of the self with the divine. All yogic systems are aimed at nurturing the body through breath and posture and cultivating the mind through meditation.

zinc
Essential mineral, found in almost every cell, that stimulates the activity of approximately 100 enzymes, which are substances that promote the body's biochemical reactions. Zinc supports a healthy immune system, is needed for wound healing, helps maintain sense of taste and smell, and is essential for DNA synthesis. Zinc also supports normal growth and development during pregnancy, childhood, and adolescence. Clinical trials are ongoing to test the use of supplemental zinc on the effects of the common cold.

Common Drugs and Their Uses*

BY GENERIC NAME

The following is a list of common generic drugs with the brand name(s) in parentheses. An explanation of the use of each drug is given. Starting on page 228, brand (or trade) names for these drugs are listed alphabetically.

GENERIC NAME (BRAND NAME)	EXPLANATION OF USE
acarbose (Precose)	Antidiabetic (type 2 diabetes)/alpha-glucosidase inhibitor
acetaminophen (Tylenol)	Analgesic/mild
acyclovir (Zovirax)	Antiviral
adalimumab (Humira)	Gastrointestinal/ anti-TNF
albuterol (Proventil, Ventolin)	Bronchodilator
alendronate (Fosamax)	Antiosteoporosis/ bisphosphonate
alprazolam (Xanax)	Tranquilizer/minor/ benzodiazepine
aluminum antacid (Rolaids)	GI/antacid
aluminum magnesium antacid (Gaviscon)	GI/antacid
amiodarone (Cordarone)	Cardiovascular/ antiarrhythmic

*From Chabner DE: The Language of Medicine, 9th ed. Philadelphia, Saunders, 2011.

COMMON DRUGS AND THEIR USES
(Continued)

GENERIC NAME (BRAND NAME)	EXPLANATION OF USE
amlodipine (Norvasc)	Cardiovascular/calcium antagonist
amoxicillin trihydrate (Amoxil, Trimox)	Antibiotic/penicillin
amoxicillin clavulanate (Augmentin)	Antibiotic/penicillin
anastrozole (Arimidex)	Endocrine/aromatase inhibitor
aripiprazole (Abilify)	Tranquilizer/major
aspirin (Anacin, Ascriptin, Excedrin)	Analgesic/NSAID
atenolol (Tenormin)	Cardiovascular/beta-blocker
atorvastatin (Lipitor)	Cardiovascular/cholesterol-lowering
azithromycin (Zithromax)	Antibiotic/erythromycin class
budesonide (Pulmicort)	Respiratory/steroid inhaler
buspirone (BuSpar)	Tranquilizer/minor
butabarbital (Butisol)	Sedative-hypnotic
caffeine	Stimulant
calcitonin (Cibacalcin)	Endocrine/thyroid
carbamazepine (Tegretol)	Anticonvulsant
cefprozil (Cefzil)	Antibiotic/cephalosporin
ceftazidime (Fortaz)	Antibiotic/cephalosporin
cefuroxime axetil (Ceftin)	Antibiotic/cephalosporin
celecoxib (Celebrex)	Analgesic/NSAID
cephalexin (Keflex)	Antibiotic/cephalosporin
certolizumab pegol (Cimzia)	Gastrointestinal/anti-TNF
cetirizine (Zyrtec)	Antihistamine

COMMON DRUGS AND THEIR USES
(Continued)

GENERIC NAME (BRAND NAME)	EXPLANATION OF USE
chlorpheniramine maleate (Chlor-Trimeton)	Antihistamine
chlorpromazine (Thorazine)	Tranquilizer, major/ phenothiazine
cholestyramine (Questran)	Cardiovascular/ cholesterol-binding
cimetidine (Tagamet)	GI/antiulcer/anti-GERD
ciprofloxacin (Cipro)	Antibiotic/quinolone
clarithromycin (Biaxin)	Antibiotic/erythromycin class
clopidogrel bisulfate (Plavix)	Antiplatelet
clotrimazole (Lotrimin, Mycelex)	Antifungal
codeine	Analgesic/narcotic
colestipol (Colestid)	Cardiovascular/ cholesterol-binding
dalteparin (Fragmin)	Anticoagulant
dexamethasone (Decadron)	Respiratory/steroid, intravenous or oral
dextroamphetamine sulfate (Dexedrine)	Stimulant
diazepam (Valium)	Tranquilizer/minor/ benzodiazepine
diclofenac sodium (Voltaren)	Analgesic/NSAID
digoxin (Lanoxin)	Cardiovascular/ anti-CHF
diltiazem (Cardizem CD)	Cardiovascular/calcium antagonist
diphenhydramine (Benadryl)	Antihistamine
diphenoxylate + atropine (Lomotil)	GI/antidiarrheal

COMMON DRUGS AND THEIR USES
(Continued)

GENERIC NAME (BRAND NAME)	EXPLANATION OF USE
donepezil (Aricept)	Anti-Alzheimer disease
doxycycline	Antibiotic/tetracycline
econazole, topical (Spectazole)	Antifungal
efavirenz (Sustiva)	Anti-HIV
enalapril maleate (Vasotec)	Cardiovascular ACE inhibitor
enoxaparin sodium (Lovenox)	Anticoagulant
epinephrine	Bronchodilator
erythromycin (Ery-Tab)	Antibiotic/erythromycin
escitalopram (Lexapro)	Antidepressant
estrogen (Premarin, Prempro, Estradiol)	Endocrine/estrogen
etanercept (Enbrel)	Gastrointestinal/ anti-TNF
ethambutol (Myambutol)	Antitubercular
ether	Anesthetic/general
famotidine (Pepcid)	GI/antiulcer/ anti-GERD
felbamate (Felbatol)	Anticonvulsant
fexofenadine (Allegra)	Antihistamine
fluconazole (Diflucan)	Antifungal
flunisolide (AeroBid)	Respiratory/steroid inhaler
fluoxymesterone (Halotestin)	Endocrine/androgen
flutamide (Eulexin)	Endocrine/ antiandrogen
fluticasone propionate (Flovent)	Respiratory/steroid inhaler
formoterol (Foradil)	Bronchodilator
formoterol + budesonide (Symbicort)	Bronchodilator

COMMON DRUGS AND THEIR USES
(Continued)

GENERIC NAME (BRAND NAME)	EXPLANATION OF USE
fulvestrant (Faslodex)	Endocrine/aromatase inhibitor
furosemide (Lasix)	Cardiovascular/diuretic
gabapentin (Neurontin)	Anticonvulsant
glipizide (Glucotrol XL)	Antidiabetic (type 2 diabetes)/sulfonylurea
glyburide	Antidiabetic (type 2 diabetes)/sulfonylurea
goserelin (Zoladex)	Endocrine/ antiandrogen
haloperidol (Haldol)	Tranquilizer/major
halothane (Fluothane)	Anesthetic/general
hydrochlorothiazide (HydroDiuril)	Cardiovascular/diuretic
hydrocodone w/APAP (Lortab, Vicodin)	Analgesic/narcotic
hydromorphone (Dilaudid)	Analgesic/narcotic
ibuprofen (Motrin, Advil)	Analgesic/NSAID
ibutilide (Corvert)	Antiarrhythmic
indinavir (Crixivan)	Antiviral/protease inhibitor/anti-HIV
infliximab (Remicade)	Gastrointestinal/ anti-TNF
insulin aspart (NovoLog)	Antidiabetic (type 1 diabetes)
insulin detemir (Levemir)	Antidiabetic (type 1 diabetes)
insulin glargine (Lantus)	Antidiabetic (type 1 diabetes)
insulin glulisine (Apidra)	Antidiabetic (type 1 diabetes)

COMMON DRUGS AND THEIR USES
(Continued)

GENERIC NAME (BRAND NAME)	EXPLANATION OF USE
insulin lispro (Humalog)	Antidiabetic (type 1 diabetes)
insulin NPH (Humulin N)	Antidiabetic (type 1 diabetes)
insulin regular (Humulin R)	Antidiabetic (type 1 diabetes)
insulin zinc suspension (Ultralente)	Antidiabetic (type 1 diabetes)
interferon alfa-n1 (Wellferon)	Antiviral/anti-cancer drug
ipratropium bromide + albuterol (Combivent)	Bronchodilator
irbesartan (Avapro)	Cardiovascular/ angiotensin II receptor antagonist
isoniazid *or* INH (Nydrazid)	Antitubercular
itraconazole (Sporanox)	Antifungal
ketorolac (Toradol)	Analgesic/NSAID
lamivudine (Epivir)	Antiviral/reverse transcriptase inhibitor/anti-HIV
lansoprazole (Prevacid)	GI/antiulcer/anti-GERD
lepirudin (Refludan)	Anticoagulant
letrozole (Femara)	Endocrine/aromatase inhibitor
leuprolide (Lupron)	Endocrine/antiandrogen
levalbuterol (Xopenex)	Bronchodilator
levofloxacin (Levaquin)	Antibiotic
levothyroxine (Levoxyl, Levothroid, Synthroid)	Endocrine/thyroid hormone
lidocaine (Xylocaine)	Anesthetic/local

COMMON DRUGS AND THEIR USES
(Continued)

GENERIC NAME (BRAND NAME)	EXPLANATION OF USE
lidocaine + prilocaine (EMLA)	Anesthetic/local
liothyronine (Cytomel)	Endocrine/thyroid hormone
liotrix (Thyrolar)	Endocrine/thyroid hormone
lisinopril (Prinivil, Zestril)	Cardiovascular/ACE inhibitor
lithium carbonate (Eskalith)	Tranquilizer/major
loperamide (Imodium)	GI/antidiarrheal
loratadine (Claritin)	Antihistamine
lorazepam (Ativan)	Tranquilizer/minor/ benzodiazepine
losartan (Cozaar)	Cardiovascular/ angiotensin II receptor antagonist
lovastatin (Mevacor)	Cardiovascular/ cholesterol-lowering
magnesium antacid (milk of magnesia)	GI/antacid
meclizine (Antivert)	Antihistamine
medroxyprogesterone acetate (Cycrin, Provera)	Endocrine/progestin
megestrol (Megace)	Endocrine/progestin
memantine (Namenda)	Anti-Alzheimer disease
meperidine (Demerol)	Analgesic/narcotic
metaproterenol (Alupent)	Bronchodilator
metformin (Glucophage)	Antidiabetic (type 2 diabetes)/biguanide
methaqualone (Quaalude)	Sedative-hypnotic

COMMON DRUGS AND THEIR USES
(Continued)

GENERIC NAME (BRAND NAME)	EXPLANATION OF USE
methylphenidate (Ritalin)	Stimulant
methylprednisolone (Medrol)	Respiratory/steroid, intravenous or oral
methyltestosterone (Virilon)	Endocrine/androgen
metoclopramide (Reglan)	GI/antinauseant
metoprolol (Lopressor, Toprol-XL)	Cardiovascular/ beta-blocker
miconazole (Monistat)	Antifungal
midazolam (Versed)	Sedative-hypnotic
modafinil (Provigil)	Stimulant/sleep antagonist
mometasone (Asmanex)	Respiratory/inhaler
montelukast sodium (Singulair)	Respiratory/leukotriene modifier
nafcillin (Unipen)	Antibiotic/penicillin
naproxen (Naprosyn)	Analgesic/NSAID
nifedipine (Adalat CC, Procardia)	Cardiovascular/calcium antagonist
nilutamide (Casodex)	Endocrine/antiandrogen
nitroglycerin	Cardiovascular/ antianginal
nitrous oxide	Anesthetic/general
nystatin (Nilstat)	Antifungal
octreotide (Sandostatin)	Endocrine/growth
ofloxacin (Floxin)	Antibiotic/quinolone
olanzapine (Zyprexa)	Tranquilizer/major/ antipsychotic
omeprazole (Prilosec)	GI/antiulcer/anti-GERD
ondansetron (Zofran)	GI/antinauseant

COMMON DRUGS AND THEIR USES
(Continued)

GENERIC NAME (BRAND NAME)	EXPLANATION OF USE
oxacillin (Bactocill)	Antibiotic/penicillin
oxycodone (OxyContin, Roxicodone)	Analgesic/narcotic
oxycodone w/APAP (Roxicet, Endocet, Percocet)	Analgesic/narcotic
pamidronate disodium (Aredia)	Anti-osteoporosis/bisphosphonate
paregoric	GI/antidiarrheal
phenobarbital (Luminal)	Sedative-hypnotic/anticonvulsant
phenytoin sodium (Dilantin)	Anticonvulsant
pioglitazone (Actos)	Antidiabetic (type 2 diabetes)
pirbuterol (Maxair)	Bronchodilator
pravastatin (Pravachol)	Cardiovascular/cholesterol-lowering
prednisone	Respiratory/steroid, intravenous or oral
promethazine (Phenergan)	Antihistamine
procaine (Novocain)	Anesthetic/local
prochlorperazine maleate (Compazine)	GI/antinauseant
propoxyphene (Darvon)	Analgesic/narcotic
propranolol (Inderal)	Cardiovascular/beta-blocker
quinapril (Accupril)	Cardiovascular/ACE inhibitor
raloxifene (Evista)	Endocrine/SERM/antiosteoporosis
ramipril (Altace)	Cardiovascular/ACE inhibitor

COMMON DRUGS AND THEIR USES
(Continued)

GENERIC NAME (BRAND NAME)	EXPLANATION OF USE
ranitidine (Zantac)	GI/antiulcer/anti-GERD
repaglinide (Prandin)	Antidiabetic (type 2 diabetes)/meglitinide
rifampin (Rifadin)	Antitubercular
risperidone (Risperdal)	Tranquilizer/major
rosiglitazone (Avandia)	Antidiabetic (type 2 diabetes)
rosuvastatin calcium (Crestor)	Cholesterol-lowering statin
salmeterol (Serevent)	Bronchodilator
salmeterol + fluticasone (Advair)	Corticosteroid anti-inflammatory–bronchodilator combination
simvastatin (Zocor)	Cardiovascular/cholesterol-lowering
sotalol (Betapace)	Cardiovascular/beta-blocker
spironolactone (Aldactone)	Cardiovascular/diuretic
sulfamethoxazole + trimethoprim (Bactrim)	Antibiotic/sulfonamide-antibacterial combination
sulfisoxazole (Gantrisin)	Antibiotic/sulfonamide
tamoxifen (Nolvadex)	Endocrine/SERM
temazepam (Restoril)	Sedative-hypnotic/benzodiazepine
terbinafine (Lamisil)	Antifungal
teriparatide (Forteo)	Endocrine/parathyroid
tetracycline (Sumycin, Terramycin)	Antibiotic/tetracycline
theophylline (Theo-Dur)	Bronchodilator

COMMON DRUGS AND THEIR USES
(Continued)

GENERIC NAME (BRAND NAME)	EXPLANATION OF USE
thiopental (Pentothal)	Anesthetic/general
thioridazine (Mellaril)	Tranquilizer/major/phenothiazine
tiotropium (Spiriva)	Bronchodilator
tissue plasminogen activator or tPA	Anticoagulant
tramadol (Ultram)	Analgesic/narcotic
triamcinolone (Azmacort)	Respiratory/steroid inhaler
triamterene (Dyazide)	Cardiovascular/diuretic
triazolam (Halcion)	Sedative-hypnotic/benzodiazepine
trifluoperazine (Stelazine)	Tranquilizer/major/phenothiazine
valdecoxib (Bextra)	Analgesic/NSAID
valproic acid (Depakote)	Anticonvulsant
warfarin (Coumadin)	Anticoagulant
zafirlukast (Accolate)	Respiratory/leukotriene modifier
zidovudine or AZT (Retrovir)	Antiviral/reverse transcriptase inhibitor/anti-HIV
zidovudine + lamivudine (Combivir)	Anti-HIV
zileuton (Zyflo)	Respiratory/leukotriene modifier
zoledronic acid (Zometa)	Antiosteoporosis/bisphosphonate
zolpidem tartrate (Ambien)	Sedative-hypnotic

BY BRAND NAME

The following is the list of common drugs by brand name with generic names in parentheses.

BRAND NAME (GENERIC NAME)	EXPLANATION OF USE
Abilify (aripiprazole)	Tranquilizer/major
Accolate (zafirlukast)	Respiratory/ leukotriene modifier
Accupril (quinapril)	Cardiovascular/ACE inhibitor
Actos (pioglitazone)	Antidiabetic (type 2 diabetes)
Adalat CC (nifedipine)	Cardiovascular/ calcium antagonist
Advair (salmeterol + fluticasone)	Corticosteroid anti-inflammatory–bronchodilator combination
Advil (ibuprofen)	Analgesic/NSAID
AeroBid (flunisolide)	Respiratory/steroid inhaler
Aldactone (spironolactone)	Cardiovascular/ diuretic
Allegra (fexofenadine)	Antihistamine
Altace (ramipril)	Cardiovascular/ACE inhibitor
Alupent (metaproterenol)	Bronchodilator
Ambien (zolpidem tartrate)	Sedative-hypnotic
Amoxil (amoxicillin trihydrate)	Antibiotic/penicillin
Anacin (aspirin)	Analgesic/NSAID
Antivert (meclizine)	Antihistamine
Apidra (insulin glulisine)	Antidiabetic (type 1 diabetes)
Aredia (pamidronate disodium)	Anti-osteoporosis/ bisphosphonate
Aricept (donepezil)	Anti-Alzheimer disease

COMMON DRUGS AND THEIR USES
(Continued)

BRAND NAME (GENERIC NAME)	EXPLANATION OF USE
Arimidex (anastrozole)	Endocrine/aromatase inhibitor
Ascriptin (aspirin)	Analgesic/NSAID
Asmanex (mometasone)	Respiratory/inhaler
Ativan (lorazepam)	Tranquilizer/minor/ benzodiazepine
Augmentin (amoxicillin clavulanate)	Antibiotic/penicillin
Avandia (rosiglitazone)	Antidiabetic (type 2 diabetes)
Avapro (irbesartan)	Cardiovascular/ angiotensin II receptor antagonist
Azmacort (triamcinolone)	Respiratory/steroid inhaler
Bactocill (oxacillin)	Antibiotic/penicillin
Bactrim (sulfamethoxazole + trimethoprim)	Antibiotic/ sulfonamide- antibacterial combination
Benadryl (diphenhydramine)	Antihistamine
Betapace (sotalol)	Cardiovascular/ beta-blocker
Bextra (valdecoxib)	Analgesic/NSAID
Biaxin (clarithromycin)	Antibiotic/ erythromycin class
BuSpar (buspirone)	Tranquilizer/minor
Butisol (butabarbital)	Sedative-hypnotic
caffeine	Stimulant
Cardizem CD (diltiazem)	Cardiovascular/ calcium antagonist
Casodex (nilutamide)	Endocrine/ antiandrogen
Ceftin (cefuroxime axetil)	Antibiotic/ cephalosporin

COMMON DRUGS AND THEIR USES
(Continued)

BRAND NAME (GENERIC NAME)	EXPLANATION OF USE
Cefzil (cefprozil)	Antibiotic/cephalosporin
Celebrex (celecoxib)	Analgesic/NSAID
Chlor-Trimeton (chlorpheniramine maleate)	Antihistamine
Cibacalcin (calcitonin)	Endocrine/thyroid
Cimzia (certolizumab pegol)	Gastrointestinal/anti-TNF
Cipro (ciprofloxacin)	Antibiotic/quinolone
Claritin (loratadine)	Antihistamine
codeine	Analgesic/narcotic
Colestid (colestipol)	Cardiovascular/cholesterol-binding
Combivent (ipratropium bromide + albuterol)	Bronchodilator
Combivir (zidovudine + lamivudine)	Anti-HIV
Compazine (prochlorperazine maleate)	GI/antinauseant
Cordarone (amiodarone)	Cardiovascular/antiarrhythmic
Corvert (ibutilide)	Antiarrhythmic
Coumadin (warfarin)	Anticoagulant
Cozaar (losartan)	Cardiovascular/angiotensin II receptor antagonist
Crestor (rosuvastatin calcium)	Cholesterol-lowering statin
Crixivan (indinavir)	Antiviral/protease inhibitor/anti-HIV
Cycrin (medroxyprogesterone acetate)	Endocrine/progestin
Cytomel (liothyronine)	Endocrine/thyroid hormone

COMMON DRUGS AND THEIR USES
(Continued)

BRAND NAME (GENERIC NAME)	EXPLANATION OF USE
Darvon (propoxyphene)	Analgesic/narcotic
Decadron (dexamethasone)	Respiratory/steroid, intravenous or oral
Demerol (meperidine)	Analgesic/narcotic
Depakote (valproic acid)	Anticonvulsant
Dexedrine (dextroamphetamine sulfate)	Stimulant
Diflucan (fluconazole)	Antifungal
Dilantin (phenytoin sodium)	Anticonvulsant
Dilaudid (hydromorphone)	Analgesic/narcotic
doxycycline	Antibiotic/tetracycline
Dyazide (triamterene)	Cardiovascular/diuretic
EMLA (lidocaine + prilocaine)	Anesthetic/local
Enbrel (etanercept)	Gastrointestinal/anti-TNF
Endocet (oxycodone w/APAP)	Analgesic/narcotic
epinephrine	Bronchodilator
Epivir (lamivudine)	Antiviral/reverse transcriptase inhibitor/anti-HIV
Ery-Tab (erythromycin)	Antibiotic/erythromycin
Eskalith (lithium carbonate)	Tranquilizer/major
Estradiol (estrogen)	Endocrine/estrogen
ether	Anesthetic/general
Eulexin (flutamide)	Endocrine/antiandrogen

COMMON DRUGS AND THEIR USES
(Continued)

BRAND NAME (GENERIC NAME)	EXPLANATION OF USE
Evista (raloxifene)	Endocrine/SERM/ antiosteoporosis
Excedrin (aspirin)	Analgesic/NSAID
Faslodex (fulvestrant)	Endocrine/aromatase inhibitor
Felbatol (felbamate)	Anticonvulsant
Femara (letrozole)	Endocrine/aromatase inhibitor
Flovent (fluticasone propionate)	Respiratory/steroid inhaler
Floxin (ofloxacin)	Antibiotic/quinolone
Fluothane (halothane)	Anesthetic/general
Foradil (formoterol)	Bronchodilator
Fortaz (ceftazidime)	Antibiotic/ cephalosporin
Forteo (teriparatide)	Endocrine/parathyroid
Fosamax (alendronate)	Antiosteoporosis/ bisphosphonate
Fragmin (dalteparin)	Anticoagulant
Gantrisin (sulfisoxazole)	Antibiotic/sulfonamide
Gaviscon (aluminum magnesium antacid)	GI/antacid
Glucophage (metformin)	Antidiabetic (type 2 diabetes)/ biguanide
Glucotrol XL (glipizide)	Antidiabetic (type 2 diabetes)/ sulfonylurea
glyburide	Antidiabetic (type 2 diabetes)/ sulfonylurea
Halcion (triazolam)	Sedative-hypnotic/ benzodiazepine
Haldol (haloperidol)	Tranquilizer/major

COMMON DRUGS AND THEIR USES
(Continued)

BRAND NAME (GENERIC NAME)	EXPLANATION OF USE
Halotestin (fluoxymesterone)	Endocrine/androgen
Humalog (insulin lispro)	Antidiabetic (type 1 diabetes)
Humira (adalimumab)	Gastrointestinal/ anti-TNF
Humulin N (insulin NPH)	Antidiabetic (type 1 diabetes)
Humulin R (insulin regular)	Antidiabetic (type 1 diabetes)
HydroDiuril (hydrochlorothiazide)	Cardiovascular/ diuretic
Imodium (loperamide)	GI/antidiarrheal
Inderal (propranolol)	Cardiovascular/ beta-blocker
Keflex (cephalexin)	Antibiotic/ cephalosporin
Lamisil (terbinafine)	Antifungal
Lanoxin (digoxin)	Cardiovascular/ anti-CHF
Lantus (insulin glargine)	Antidiabetic (type 1 diabetes)
Lasix (furosemide)	Cardiovascular/ diuretic
Levaquin (levofloxacin)	Antibiotic
Levemir (insulin detemir)	Antidiabetic (type 1 diabetes)
Levothroid (levothyroxine)	Endocrine/thyroid hormone
Levoxyl (levothyroxine)	Endocrine/thyroid hormone
Lexapro (escitalopram)	Antidepressant
Lipitor (atorvastatin)	Cardiovascular/ cholesterol-lowering

COMMON DRUGS AND THEIR USES
(Continued)

BRAND NAME (GENERIC NAME)	EXPLANATION OF USE
Lomotil (diphenoxylate + atropine)	GI/antidiarrheal
Lopressor (metoprolol)	Cardiovascular/ beta-blocker
Lortab (hydrocodone w/APAP)	Analgesic/narcotic
Lotrimin (clotrimazole)	Antifungal
Lovenox (enoxaparin sodium)	Anticoagulant
Luminal (phenobarbital)	Sedative-hypnotic/ anticonvulsant
Lupron (leuprolide)	Endocrine/ antiandrogen
Maxair (pirbuterol)	Bronchodilator
Medrol (methylprednisolone)	Respiratory/steroid, intravenous or oral
Megace (megestrol)	Endocrine/progestin
Mellaril (thioridazine)	Tranquilizer/major/ phenothiazine
Mevacor (lovastatin)	Cardiovascular/ cholesterol-lowering
milk of magnesia (magnesium antacid)	GI/antacid
Monistat (miconazole)	Antifungal
Motrin (ibuprofen)	Analgesic/NSAID
Myambutol (ethambutol)	Antitubercular
Mycelex (clotrimazole)	Antifungal
Namenda (memantine)	Anti-Alzheimer disease
Naprosyn (naproxen)	Analgesic/NSAID
Neurontin (gabapentin)	Anticonvulsant
Nilstat (nystatin)	Antifungal
nitroglycerin	Cardiovascular/ antianginal
nitrous oxide	Anesthetic/general

COMMON DRUGS AND THEIR USES
(Continued)

BRAND NAME (GENERIC NAME)	EXPLANATION OF USE
Nolvadex (tamoxifen)	Endocrine/SERM
Norvasc (amlodipine)	Cardiovascular/ calcium antagonist
Novocain (procaine)	Anesthetic/local
NovoLog (insulin aspart)	Antidiabetic (type 1 diabetes)
Nydrazid (isoniazid *or* INH)	Antitubercular
OxyContin (oxycodone)	Analgesic/narcotic
paregoric	GI/antidiarrheal
Pentothal (thiopental)	Anesthetic/general
Pepcid (famotidine)	GI/antiulcer/ anti-GERD
Percocet (oxycodone w/APAP)	Analgesic/narcotic
Phenergan (promethazine)	Antihistamine
Plavix (clopidogrel bisulfate)	Antiplatelet
Prandin (repaglinide)	Antidiabetic (type 2 diabetes)/ meglitinide
Pravachol (pravastatin)	Cardiovascular/ cholesterol-lowering
Precose (acarbose)	Antidiabetic (type 2 diabetes)/ alpha-glucosidase inhibitor
prednisone	Respiratory/steroid, intravenous or oral
Premarin (estrogen)	Endocrine/estrogen
Prempro (estrogen)	Endocrine/estrogen
Prevacid (lansoprazole)	GI/antiulcer/ anti-GERD

COMMON DRUGS AND THEIR USES
(Continued)

BRAND NAME (GENERIC NAME)	EXPLANATION OF USE
Prilosec (omeprazole)	GI/antiulcer/anti-GERD
Prinivil (lisinopril)	Cardiovascular/ACE inhibitor
Procardia (nifedipine)	Cardiovascular/calcium antagonist
Proventil (albuterol)	Bronchodilator
Provera (medroxyprogesterone acetate)	Endocrine/progestin
Provigil (modafinil)	Stimulant/sleep antagonist
Pulmicort (budesonide)	Respiratory/steroid inhaler
Quaalude (methaqualone)	Sedative-hypnotic
Questran (cholestyramine)	Cardiovascular/cholesterol-binding
Refludan (lepirudin)	Anticoagulant
Reglan (metoclopramide)	GI/antinauseant
Remicade (infliximab)	Gastrointestinal/anti-TNF
Restoril (temazepam)	Sedative-hypnotic/benzodiazepine
Retrovir (zidovudine or AZT)	Antiviral/reverse transcriptase inhibitor/anti-HIV
Rifadin (rifampin)	Antitubercular
Risperdal (risperidone)	Tranquilizer/major
Ritalin (methylphenidate)	Stimulant
Rolaids (aluminum antacid)	GI/antacid

COMMON DRUGS AND THEIR USES
(Continued)

BRAND NAME (GENERIC NAME)	EXPLANATION OF USE
Roxicet (oxycodone w/APAP)	Analgesic/narcotic
Roxicodone (oxycodone)	Analgesic/narcotic
Sandostatin (octreotide)	Endocrine/growth
Serevent (salmeterol)	Bronchodilator
Singulair (montelukast sodium)	Respiratory/ leukotriene modifier
Spectazole (econazole, topical)	Antifungal
Spiriva (tiotropium)	Bronchodilator
Sporanox (itraconazole)	Antifungal
Stelazine (trifluoperazine)	Tranquilizer/major/ phenothiazine
Sumycin (tetracycline)	Antibiotic/tetracycline
Sustiva (efavirenz)	Anti-HIV
Symbicort (formoterol + budesonide)	Bronchodilator
Synthroid (levothyroxine)	Endocrine/thyroid hormone
Tagamet (cimetidine)	GI/antiulcer/anti-GERD
Tegretol (carbamazepine)	Anticonvulsant
Tenormin (atenolol)	Cardiovascular/ beta-blocker
Terramycin (tetracycline)	Antibiotic/tetracycline
Theo-Dur (theophylline)	Bronchodilator
Thorazine (chlorpromazine)	Tranquilizer, major/ phenothiazine
Thyrolar (liotrix)	Endocrine/thyroid hormone
tissue plasminogen activator or tPA	Anticoagulant

COMMON DRUGS AND THEIR USES
(Continued)

BRAND NAME (GENERIC NAME)	EXPLANATION OF USE
Toprol-XL (metoprolol)	Cardiovascular/beta-blocker
Toradol (ketorolac)	Analgesic/NSAID
Trimox (amoxicillin trihydrate)	Antibiotic/penicillin
Tylenol (acetaminophen)	Analgesic/mild
Ultralente (insulin zinc suspension)	Antidiabetic (type 1 diabetes)
Ultram (tramadol)	Analgesic/narcotic
Unipen (nafcillin)	Antibiotic/penicillin
Valium (diazepam)	Tranquilizer/minor/benzodiazepine
Vasotec (enalapril maleate)	Cardiovascular ACE inhibitor
Ventolin (albuterol)	Bronchodilator
Versed (midazolam)	Sedative-hypnotic
Vicodin (hydrocodone w/APAP)	Analgesic/narcotic
Virilon (methyltestosterone)	Endocrine/androgen
Voltaren (diclofenac sodium)	Analgesic/NSAID
Wellferon (interferon alfa-n1)	Antiviral/anti-cancer drug
Xanax (alprazolam)	Tranquilizer/minor/benzodiazepine
Xopenex (levalbuterol)	Bronchodilator
Xylocaine (lidocaine)	Anesthetic/local
Zantac (ranitidine)	GI/antiulcer/anti-GERD
Zestril (lisinopril)	Cardiovascular/ACE inhibitor

COMMON DRUGS AND THEIR USES
(Continued)

BRAND NAME (GENERIC NAME)	EXPLANATION OF USE
Zithromax (azithromycin)	Antibiotic/ erythromycin class
Zocor (simvastatin)	Cardiovascular/ cholesterol-lowering
Zofran (ondansetron)	GI/antinauseant
Zoladex (goserelin)	Endocrine/ antiandrogen
Zometa (zoledronic acid)	Antiosteoporosis/ bisphosphonate
Zovirax (acyclovir)	Antiviral
Zyflo (zileuton)	Respiratory/ leukotriene modifier
Zyprexa (olanzapine)	Tranquilizer/major/ antipsychotic
Zyrtec (cetirizine)	Antihistamine

Major Diagnostic Categories and Diagnosis-Related Groups (DRGs)*

There are 25 major diagnostic categories into which diagnoses are grouped. They are separated according to body system or medical specialty. These categories are one component of the Diagnostic-Related Groups (DRGs) that are used in medical coding.

MAJOR DIAGNOSTIC CATEGORIES (MDC)[†]

DIAGNOSTIC CATEGORY	GROUP DESCRIPTION
1	Diseases and disorders of the nervous system
2	Diseases and disorders of the eye
3	Diseases and disorders of the ear, nose, mouth, and throat
4	Diseases and disorders of the respiratory system
5	Diseases and disorders of the circulatory system
6	Diseases and disorders of the digestive system

*Modified from Miller-Keane Encyclopedia & Dictionary of Medicine, Nursing, & Allied Health, 7th ed., revised reprint. Philadelphia, Saunders, 2005.

[†]Excerpted from *Federal Register* 67(148):50230, August 1, 2002.

MAJOR DIAGNOSTIC CATEGORIES (MDC)
(Continued)

DIAGNOSTIC CATEGORY	GROUP DESCRIPTION
7	Diseases and disorders of the hepatobiliary system and pancreas
8	Diseases and disorders of the musculoskeletal system and connective tissue
9	Diseases and disorders of the skin, subcutaneous tissue, and breast
10	Endocrine, nutritional, and metabolic diseases and disorders
11	Diseases and disorders of the kidney and urinary tract
12	Diseases and disorders of the male reproductive system
13	Diseases and disorders of the female reproductive system
14	Pregnancy, childbirth, and the puerperium
15	Newborns and other neonates with conditions originating in the perinatal period
16	Diseases and disorders of the blood and blood-forming organs and immunologic disorders
17	Myeloproliferative diseases and disorders and poorly differentiated neoplasms
18	Infectious and parasitic diseases (systemic or unspecified sites)
19	Mental diseases and disorders

MAJOR DIAGNOSTIC CATEGORIES (MDC)
(Continued)

DIAGNOSTIC CATEGORY	GROUP DESCRIPTION
20	Alcohol/drug use and alcohol/drug-induced organic mental disorders
21	Injuries, poisonings, and toxic effects of drugs
22	Burns
23	Factors influencing health status and other contacts with health services
24	Multiple significant trauma
25	Human immunodeficiency virus infections

DIAGNOSIS-RELATED GROUPS (DRGs)*

Please note the following abbreviations used in this section: AICD, automated implantable cardioverter-defibrillator; AMA, against medical advice; AMI, acute myocardial infarction; CC, comorbidity/complications; CDE, complete diagnostic evaluation; D & C, dilatation & curettage; DIS, disease; Fx, fracture; GI, gastrointestinal; GNR, generator procedure; HRT, heart; IM, implant; OR, operating room; PTCA, percutaneous transluminal coronary angioplasty; SHK, shock; TIA, transient ischemic attack; URI, upper respiratory infection.

DRG	MDC	TYPE	DESCRIPTION
1	01	Surg	Craniotomy age >17 except for trauma
2	01	Surg	Craniotomy for trauma age >17

---

*Excerpted from *Federal Register* 67(148):50230, August 1, 2002.

DIAGNOSIS-RELATED GROUPS (DRGs)
(Continued)

DRG	MDC	TYPE	DESCRIPTION
3	01	Surg	Craniotomy age 0–17
4	01	Surg	Spinal procedures
5	01	Surg	Extracranial vascular procedures
6	01	Surg	Carpal tunnel release
7	01	Surg	Peripheral and cranial nerve and other nerve syst proc w CC
8	01	Surg	Peripheral and cranial nerve and other nerve syst proc w/o CC
9	01	Med	Spinal disorders and injuries
10	01	Med	Nervous system neoplasms w CC
11	01	Med	Nervous system neoplasms w/o CC
12	01	Med	Degenerative nervous system disorders
13	01	Med	Multiple sclerosis and cerebellar ataxia
14	01	Med	Specific cerebrovascular disorders except TIA
15	01	Med	Transient ischemic attack and precerebral occlusions
16	01	Med	Nonspecific cerebrovascular disorders w CC
17	01	Med	Nonspecific cerebrovascular disorders w/o CC

DIAGNOSIS-RELATED GROUPS (DRGs)
(Continued)

DRG	MDC	TYPE	DESCRIPTION
18	01	Med	Cranial and peripheral nerve disorders w CC
19	01	Med	Cranial and peripheral nerve disorders w/o CC
20	01	Med	Nervous system infection except viral meningitis
21	01	Med	Viral meningitis
22	01	Med	Hypertensive encephalopathy
23	01	Med	Nontraumatic stupor and coma
24	01	Med	Seizure and headache age >17 w CC
25	01	Med	Seizure and headache age >17 w/o CC
26	01	Med	Seizure and headache age 0–17
27	01	Med	Traumatic stupor and coma, coma >1 hr
28	01	Med	Traumatic stupor and coma, coma <1 hr age >17 w CC
29	01	Med	Traumatic stupor and coma, coma <1 hr age >17 w/o CC
30	01	Med	Traumatic stupor and coma, coma <1 hr age 0–17
31	01	Med	Concussion age >17 w CC
32	01	Med	Concussion age >17 w/o CC
33	01	Med	Concussion age 0–17

DIAGNOSIS-RELATED GROUPS (DRGs)
(Continued)

DRG	MDC	TYPE	DESCRIPTION
34	01	Med	Other disorders of nervous system w CC
35	01	Med	Other disorders of nervous system w/o CC
36	02	Surg	Retinal procedures
37	02	Surg	Orbital procedures
38	02	Surg	Primary iris procedures
39	02	Surg	Lens procedures with or without vitrectomy
40	02	Surg	Extraocular procedures except orbit age >17
41	02	Surg	Extraocular procedures except orbit age 0–17
42	02	Surg	Intraocular procedures except retina, iris and lens
43	02	Med	Hyphema
44	02	Med	Acute major eye infections
45	02	Med	Neurological eye disorders
46	02	Med	Other disorders of the eye age >17 w CC
47	02	Med	Other disorders of the eye age >17 w/o CC
48	02	Med	Other disorders of the eye age 0–17
49	03	Surg	Major head and neck procedures
50	03	Surg	Sialoadenectomy
51	03	Surg	Salivary gland procedures except sialoadenectomy

DIAGNOSIS-RELATED GROUPS (DRGs)
(Continued)

DRG	MDC	TYPE	DESCRIPTION
52	03	Surg	Cleft lip and palate repair
53	03	Surg	Sinus and mastoid procedures age >17
54	03	Surg	Sinus and mastoid procedures age 0–17
55	03	Surg	Miscellaneous ear, nose, mouth and throat procedures
56	03	Surg	Rhinoplasty
57	03	Surg	T and A proc, except tonsillectomy and/or adenoidectomy only, age >17
58	03	Surg	T and A proc, except tonsillectomy and/or adenoidectomy only, age 0–17
59	03	Surg	Tonsillectomy and/or adenoidectomy only, age >17
60	03	Surg	Tonsillectomy and/or adenoidectomy only, age 0-17
61	03	Surg	Myringotomy w tube insertion age >17
62	03	Surg	Myringotomy w tube insertion age 0–17
63	03	Surg	Other ear, nose, mouth and throat O.R. procedures
64	03	Med	Ear, nose, mouth and throat malignancy

DIAGNOSIS-RELATED GROUPS (DRGs)
(Continued)

DRG	MDC	TYPE	DESCRIPTION
65	03	Med	Dysequilibrium
66	03	Med	Epistaxis
67	03	Med	Epiglottitis
68	03	Med	Otitis media and uri age >17 w CC
69	03	Med	Otitis media and uri age >17 w/o CC
70	03	Med	Otitis media and uri age 0–17
71	03	Med	Laryngotracheitis
72	03	Med	Nasal trauma and deformity
73	03	Med	Other ear, nose, mouth and throat diagnoses age >17
74	03	Med	Other ear, nose, mouth and throat diagnoses age 0–17
75	04	Surg	Major chest procedures
76	04	Surg	Other resp system OR procedures w CC
77	04	Surg	Other resp system OR procedures w/o CC
78	04	Med	Pulmonary embolism
79	04	Med	Respiratory infections and inflammations age >17 w CC
80	04	Med	Respiratory infections and inflammations age >17 w/o CC

DIAGNOSIS-RELATED GROUPS (DRGs)
(Continued)

DRG	MDC	TYPE	DESCRIPTION
81	04	Med	Respiratory infections and inflammations age 0–17
82	04	Med	Respiratory neoplasms
83	04	Med	Major chest trauma w CC
84	04	Med	Major chest trauma w/o CC
85	04	Med	Pleural effusion w CC
86	04	Med	Pleural effusion w/o CC
87	04	Med	Pulmonary edema and respiratory failure
88	04	Med	Chronic obstructive pulmonary disease
89	04	Med	Simple pneumonia and pleurisy age >17 w CC
90	04	Med	Simple pneumonia and pleurisy age >17 w/o CC
91	04	Med	Simple pneumonia and pleurisy age 0–17
92	04	Med	Interstitial lung disease w CC
93	04	Med	Interstitial lung disease w/o CC
94	04	Med	Pneumothorax w CC
95	04	Med	Pneumothorax w/o CC
96	04	Med	Bronchitis and asthma age >17 w CC
97	04	Med	Bronchitis and asthma age >17 w/o CC

DIAGNOSIS-RELATED GROUPS (DRGs)
(Continued)

DRG	MDC	TYPE	DESCRIPTION
98	04	Med	Bronchitis and asthma age 0–17
99	04	Med	Respiratory signs and symptoms w CC
100	04	Med	Respiratory signs and symptoms w/o CC
101	04	Med	Other respiratory system diagnoses w CC
102	04	Med	Other respiratory system diagnoses w/o CC
103	05	Surg	Heart transplant
104	05	Surg	Cardiac valve and other major cardiothoracic proc w cardiac cath
105	05	Surg	Cardiac valve and other major cardiothoracic proc w/o cardiac cath
106	05	Surg	Coronary bypass w PTCA
107	05	Surg	Coronary bypass w cardiac cath
108	05	Surg	Other cardiothoracic procedures
109	05	Surg	Coronary bypass w/o PTCA or cardiac cath
110	05	Surg	Major cardiovascular procedures w CC
111	05	Surg	Major cardiovascular procedures w/o CC
112	05	Surg	Percutaneous cardiovascular procedures

DIAGNOSIS-RELATED GROUPS (DRGs)
(Continued)

DRG	MDC	TYPE	DESCRIPTION
113	05	Surg	Amputation for circ system disorders except upper limb and toe
114	05	Surg	Upper limb and toe amputation for circ system disorders
115	05	Surg	Perm card pacem impl w AMI, HRT fail or SHK, or AICD lead or GNR
116	05	Surg	Oth perm card pacemak impl or PTCA w coronary artery stent IM
117	05	Surg	Cardiac pacemaker revision except device replacement
118	05	Surg	Cardiac pacemaker device replacement
119	05	Surg	Vein ligation and stripping
120	05	Surg	Other circulatory system O.R. procedures
121	05	Med	Circulatory disorders w AMI and major comp, discharged alive
122	05	Med	Circulatory disorders w AMI w/o major comp, discharged alive
123	05	Med	Circulatory disorders w AMI, expired
124	05	Med	Circulatory disorders except AMI, w card cath and complex diag

DIAGNOSIS-RELATED GROUPS (DRGs)
(Continued)

DRG	MDC	TYPE	DESCRIPTION
125	05	Med	Circulatory disorders except AMI, w card cath w/o complex diag
126	05	Med	Acute and subacute endocarditis
127	05	Med	Heart failure and shock
128	05	Med	Deep vein thrombophlebitis
129	05	Med	Cardiac arrest, unexplained
130	05	Med	Peripheral vascular disorders w CC
131	05	Med	Peripheral vascular disorders w/o CC
132	05	Med	Atherosclerosis w CC
133	05	Med	Atherosclerosis w/o CC
134	05	Med	Hypertension
135	05	Med	Cardiac congenital and valvular disorders age >17 w CC
136	05	Med	Cardiac congenital and valvular disorders age >17 w/o CC
137	05	Med	Cardiac congenital and valvular disorders age 0–17
138	05	Med	Cardiac arrhythmia and conduction disorders w CC
139	05	Med	Cardiac arrhythmia and conduction disorders w/o CC

DIAGNOSIS-RELATED GROUPS (DRGs)
(Continued)

DRG	MDC	TYPE	DESCRIPTION
140	05	Med	Angina pectoris
141	05	Med	Syncope and collapse w CC
142	05	Med	Syncope and collapse w/o CC
143	05	Med	Chest pain
144	05	Med	Other circulatory system diagnoses w CC
145	05	Med	Other circulatory system diagnoses w/o CC
146	06	Surg	Rectal resection w CC
147	06	Surg	Rectal resection w/o CC
148	06	Surg	Major small and large bowel procedures w CC
149	06	Surg	Major small and large bowel procedures w/o CC
150	06	Surg	Peritoneal adhesiolysis w CC
151	06	Surg	Peritoneal adhesiolysis w/o CC
152	06	Surg	Minor small and large bowel procedures w CC
153	06	Surg	Minor small and large bowel procedures w/o CC
154	06	Surg	Stomach, esophageal and duodenal procedures age >17 w CC
155	06	Surg	Stomach, esophageal and duodenal procedures age >17 w/o CC

DIAGNOSIS-RELATED GROUPS (DRGs)
(Continued)

DRG	MDC	TYPE	DESCRIPTION
156	06	Surg	Stomach, esophageal and duodenal procedures age 0–17
157	06	Surg	Anal and stomal procedures w CC
158	06	Surg	Anal and stomal procedures w/o CC
159	06	Surg	Hernia procedures except inguinal and femoral age >17 w CC
160	06	Surg	Hernia procedures except inguinal and femoral age >17 w/o CC
161	06	Surg	Inguinal and femoral hernia procedures age >17 w CC
162	06	Surg	Inguinal and femoral hernia procedures age >17 w/o CC
163	06	Surg	Hernia procedures age 0–17
164	06	Surg	Appendectomy w complicated principal diag w CC
165	06	Surg	Appendectomy w complicated principal diag w/o CC
166	06	Surg	Appendectomy w/o complicated principal diag w CC
167	06	Surg	Appendectomy w/o complicated principal diag w/o CC
168	03	Surg	Mouth procedures w CC

DIAGNOSIS-RELATED GROUPS (DRGs)
(Continued)

DRG	MDC	TYPE	DESCRIPTION
169	03	Surg	Mouth procedures w/o CC
170	06	Surg	Other digestive system OR procedures w CC
171	06	Surg	Other digestive system OR procedures w/o CC
172	06	Med	Digestive malignancy w CC
173	06	Med	Digestive malignancy w/o CC
174	06	Med	G.I. hemorrhage w CC
175	06	Med	G.I. hemorrhage w/o CC
176	06	Med	Complicated peptic ulcer
177	06	Med	Uncomplicated peptic ulcer w CC
178	06	Med	Uncomplicated peptic ulcer w/o CC
179	06	Med	Inflammatory bowel disease
180	06	Med	GI obstruction w CC
181	06	Med	GI obstruction w/o CC
182	06	Med	Esophagitis, gastroent and misc digest disorders age >17 w CC
183	06	Med	Esophagitis, gastroent and misc digest disorders age >17 w/o CC
184	06	Med	Esophagitis, gastroent and misc digest disorders age 0–17

DIAGNOSIS-RELATED GROUPS (DRGs)
(Continued)

DRG	MDC	TYPE	DESCRIPTION
185	03	Med	Dental and oral DIS except extractions and restorations, age >17
186	03	Med	Dental and oral DIS except extractions and restorations, age 0–17
187	03	Med	Dental extraction and restorations
188	06	Med	Other digestive system diagnoses age >17 w CC
189	06	Med	Other digestive system diagnoses age >17 w/o CC
190	06	Med	Other digestive system diagnoses age 0–17
191	07	Surg	Pancreas, liver and shunt procedures w CC
192	07	Surg	Pancreas, liver and shunt procedures w/o CC
193	07	Surg	Biliary tract proc except only cholecyst w or w/o CDE w CC
194	07	Surg	Biliary tract proc except only cholecyst w or w/o CDE w/o CC
195	07	Surg	Cholecystectomy w CDE w CC
196	07	Surg	Cholecystectomy w CDE w/o CC
197	07	Surg	Cholecystectomy except by laparoscope w/o CDE w CC

DIAGNOSIS-RELATED GROUPS (DRGs)
(Continued)

DRG	MDC	TYPE	DESCRIPTION
198	07	Surg	Cholecystectomy except by laparoscope w/o CDE w/o CC
199	07	Surg	Hepatobiliary diagnostic procedure for malignancy
200	07	Surg	Hepatobiliary diagnostic procedure for non-malignancy
201	07	Surg	Other hepatobiliary or pancreas OR procedures
202	07	Med	Cirrhosis and alcoholic hepatitis
203	07	Med	Malignancy of hepatobiliary system or pancreas
204	07	Med	Disorders of pancreas except malignancy
205	07	Med	Disorders of liver except malig, cirr, alc hepa w CC
206	07	Med	Disorders of liver except malig, cirr, alc hepa w/o CC
207	07	Med	Disorders of the biliary tract w CC
208	07	Med	Disorders of the biliary tract w/o CC
209	08	Surg	Major joint and limb reattachment procedures of lower extremity
210	08	Surg	Hip and femur procedures except major joint age >17 w CC

DIAGNOSIS-RELATED GROUPS (DRGs)
(Continued)

DRG	MDC	TYPE	DESCRIPTION
211	08	Surg	Hip and femur procedures except major joint age >17 w/o CC
212	08	Surg	Hip and femur procedures except major joint age 0–17
213	08	Surg	Amputation for musculoskeletal system and conn tissue disorders
214	08	Surg	No longer valid
215	08	Surg	No longer valid
216	08	Surg	Biopsies of musculoskeletal system and connective tissue
217	08	Surg	Wnd debrid and skn grft except hand, for muscskelet and conn tiss disorders
218	08	Surg	Lower extrem and humer proc except hip, foot, femur age >17 w CC
219	08	Surg	Lower extrem and humer proc except hip, foot, femur age >17 w/o CC
220	08	Surg	Lower extrem and humer proc except hip, foot, femur age 0–17
221	08	Surg	No longer valid
222	08	Surg	No longer valid
223	08	Surg	Major shoulder/elbow proc, or other upper extremity proc, w/o CC

DIAGNOSIS-RELATED GROUPS (DRGs)
(Continued)

DRG	MDC	TYPE	DESCRIPTION
224	08	Surg	Shoulder, elbow or forearm proc, exc major joint proc, w/o CC
225	08	Surg	Foot procedures
226	08	Surg	Soft tissue procedures w CC
227	08	Surg	Soft tissue procedures w/o CC
228	08	Surg	Major thumb or joint proc, or oth hand or wrist proc w CC
229	08	Surg	Hand or wrist proc, except major joint proc, w/o CC
230	08	Surg	Local excision and removal of int fix devices of hip and femur
231	08	Surg	Local excision and removal of int fix devices except hip and femur
232	08	Surg	Arthroscopy
233	08	Surg	Other musculoskelet sys and conn tiss OR proc w CC
234	08	Surg	Other musculoskelet sys and conn tiss OR proc w/o CC
235	08	Med	Fractures of femur
236	08	Med	Fractures of hip and pelvis
237	08	Med	Sprains, strains, and dislocations of hip, pelvis and thigh
238	08	Med	Osteomyelitis

DIAGNOSIS-RELATED GROUPS (DRGs)
(Continued)

DRG	MDC	TYPE	DESCRIPTION
239	08	Med	Pathological fractures and musculoskeletal and conn tiss malignancy
240	08	Med	Connective tissue disorders w CC
241	08	Med	Connective tissue disorders w/o CC
242	08	Med	Septic arthritis
243	08	Med	Medical back problems
244	08	Med	Bone diseases and specific arthropathies w CC
245	08	Med	Bone diseases and specific arthropathies w/o CC
246	08	Med	Nonspecific arthropathies
247	08	Med	Signs and symptoms of musculoskeletal system and conn tissue
248	08	Med	Tendinitis, myositis, and bursitis
249	08	Med	Aftercare, musculoskeletal system and connective tissue
250	08	Med	Fx, sprn, strn and disl of forearm, hand, foot, age >17 w CC
251	08	Med	Fx, sprn, strn and disl of forearm, hand, foot, age >17 w/o CC
252	08	Med	Fx, sprn, strn and disl of forearm, hand, foot, age 0–17

DIAGNOSIS-RELATED GROUPS (DRGs)
(Continued)

DRG	MDC	TYPE	DESCRIPTION
253	08	Med	Fx, sprn, strn and disl of uparm, lowleg ex foot, age >17 w CC
254	08	Med	Fx, sprn, strn and disl of uparm, lowleg ex, foot age >17 w/o CC
255	08	Med	Fx, sprn, strn and disl of uparm, lowleg ex foot, age 0–17
256	08	Med	Other musculoskeletal system and connective tissue diagnoses
257	09	Surg	Total mastectomy for malignancy w CC
258	09	Surg	Total mastectomy for malignancy w/o CC
259	09	Surg	Subtotal mastectomy for malignancy w CC
260	09	Surg	Subtotal mastectomy for malignancy w/o CC
261	09	Surg	Breast proc for non-malignancy except biopsy and local excision
262	09	Surg	Breast biopsy and local excision for non-malignancy
263	09	Surg	Skin graft and/or debrid for skin ulcer or cellulitis w CC

DIAGNOSIS-RELATED GROUPS (DRGs)
(Continued)

DRG	MDC	TYPE	DESCRIPTION
264	09	Surg	Skin graft and/or debrid for skin ulcer or cellulitis w/o CC
265	09	Surg	Skin graft and/or debrid except for skin ulcer or cellulitis w CC
266	09	Surg	Skin graft and/or debrid except for skin ulcer or cellulitis w/o CC
267	09	Surg	Perianal and pilonidal procedures
268	09	Surg	Skin, subcutaneous tissue and breast plastic procedures
269	09	Surg	Other skin, subcut tiss and breast proc w CC
270	09	Surg	Other skin, subcut tiss and breast proc w/o CC
271	09	Med	Skin ulcers
272	09	Med	Major skin disorders w CC
273	09	Med	Major skin disorders w/o CC
274	09	Med	Malignant breast disorders w CC
275	09	Med	Malignant breast disorders w/o CC
276	09	Med	Non-malignant breast disorders
277	09	Med	Cellulitis age >17 w CC
278	09	Med	Cellulitis age >17 w/o CC

DIAGNOSIS-RELATED GROUPS (DRGs)
(Continued)

DRG	MDC	TYPE	DESCRIPTION
279	09	Med	Cellulitis age 0–17
280	09	Med	Trauma to the skin, subcut tiss and breast age >17 w CC
281	09	Med	Trauma to the skin, subcut tiss and breast age >17 w/o CC
282	09	Med	Trauma to the skin, subcut tiss and breast age 0–17
283	09	Med	Minor skin disorders w CC
284	09	Med	Minor skin disorders w/o CC
285	10	Surg	Amputat of lower limb for endocrine, nutrit and metabol disorder
286	10	Surg	Adrenal and pituitary procedures
287	10	Surg	Skin grafts and wound debrid for endoc, nutrit and metabol disorder
288	10	Surg	OR procedures for obesity
289	10	Surg	Parathyroid procedures
290	10	Surg	Thyroid procedures
291	10	Surg	Thyroglossal procedures
292	10	Surg	Other endocrine, nutrit and metab OR proc w CC
293	10	Surg	Other endocrine, nutrit and metab OR proc w/o CC
294	10	Med	Diabetes age >35

DIAGNOSIS-RELATED GROUPS (DRGs)
(Continued)

DRG	MDC	TYPE	DESCRIPTION
295	10	Med	Diabetes age 0–35
296	10	Med	Nutritional and misc metabolic disorders age >17 w CC
297	10	Med	Nutritional and misc metabolic disorders age >17 w/o CC
298	10	Med	Nutritional and misc metabolic disorders age 0–17
299	10	Med	Inborn errors of metabolism
300	10	Med	Endocrine disorders w CC
301	10	Med	Endocrine disorders w/o CC
302	11	Surg	Kidney transplant
303	11	Surg	Kidney, ureter and major bladder procedures for neoplasm
304	11	Surg	Kidney, ureter and major bladder proc for non-neopl w CC
305	11	Surg	Kidney, ureter and major bladder proc for non-neopl w/o CC
306	11	Surg	Prostatectomy w CC
307	11	Surg	Prostatectomy w/o CC
308	11	Surg	Minor bladder procedures w CC
309	11	Surg	Minor bladder procedures w/o CC

DIAGNOSIS-RELATED GROUPS (DRGs)
(Continued)

DRG	MDC	TYPE	DESCRIPTION
310	11	Surg	Transurethral procedures w CC
311	11	Surg	Transurethral procedures w/o CC
312	11	Surg	Urethral procedures, age >17 w CC
313	11	Surg	Urethral procedures, age >17 w/o CC
314	11	Surg	Urethral procedures, age 0–17
315	11	Surg	Other kidney and urinary tract OR procedures
316	11	Med	Renal failure
317	11	Med	Admit for renal dialysis
318	11	Med	Kidney and urinary tract neoplasms w CC
319	11	Med	Kidney and urinary tract neoplasms w/o CC
320	11	Med	Kidney and urinary tract infections age >17 w CC
321	11	Med	Kidney and urinary tract infections age >17 w/o CC
322	11	Med	Kidney and urinary tract infections age 0–17
323	11	Med	Urinary stones w CC, and/or ESW lithotripsy
324	11	Med	Urinary stones w/o CC
325	11	Med	Kidney and urinary tract signs and symptoms age >17 w CC

DIAGNOSIS-RELATED GROUPS (DRGs)
(Continued)

DRG	MDC	TYPE	DESCRIPTION
326	11	Med	Kidney and urinary tract signs and symptoms age >17 w/o CC
327	11	Med	Kidney and urinary tract signs and symptoms age 0–17
328	11	Med	Urethral stricture age >17 w CC
329	11	Med	Urethral stricture age >17 w/o CC
330	11	Med	Urethral stricture age 0–17
331	11	Med	Other kidney and urinary tract diagnoses age >17 w CC
332	11	Med	Other kidney and urinary tract diagnoses age >17 w/o CC
333	11	Med	Other kidney and urinary tract diagnoses age 0–17
334	12	Surg	Major male pelvic procedures w CC
335	12	Surg	Major male pelvic procedures w/o CC
336	12	Surg	Transurethral prostatectomy w CC
337	12	Surg	Transurethral prostatectomy w/o CC
338	12	Surg	Testes procedures, for malignancy

DIAGNOSIS-RELATED GROUPS (DRGs)
(Continued)

DRG	MDC	TYPE	DESCRIPTION
339	12	Surg	Testes procedures, non-malignancy age >17
340	12	Surg	Testes procedures, non-malignancy age 0–17
341	12	Surg	Penis procedures
342	12	Surg	Circumcision age >17
343	12	Surg	Circumcision age 0–17
344	12	Surg	Other male reproductive system OR procedures for malignancy
345	12	Surg	Other male reproductive system OR proc except for malignancy
346	12	Med	Malignancy, male reproductive system, w CC
347	12	Med	Malignancy, male reproductive system, w/o CC
348	12	Med	Benign prostatic hypertrophy w CC
349	12	Med	Benign prostatic hypertrophy w/o CC
350	12	Med	Inflammation of the male reproductive system
351	12	Med	Sterilization, male
352	12	Med	Other male reproductive system diagnoses

DIAGNOSIS-RELATED GROUPS (DRGs)
(Continued)

DRG	MDC	TYPE	DESCRIPTION
353	13	Surg	Pelvic evisceration, radical hysterectomy, and radical vulvectomy
354	13	Surg	Uterine, adnexa proc for non-ovarian/adnexal malig w CC
355	13	Surg	Uterine, adnexa proc for non-ovarian/adnexal malig w/o CC
356	13	Surg	Female reproductive system reconstructive procedures
357	13	Surg	Uterine and adnexa proc for ovarian or adnexal malignancy
358	13	Surg	Uterine and adnexa proc for non-malignancy w CC
359	13	Surg	Uterine and adnexa proc for non-malignancy w/o CC
360	13	Surg	Vagina, cervix and vulva procedures
361	13	Surg	Laparoscopy and incisional tubal interruption
362	13	Surg	Endoscopic tubal interruption
363	13	Surg	D & C, conization and radio-implant, for malignancy
364	13	Surg	D & C, conization except for malignancy
365	13	Surg	Other female reproductive system OR procedures

DIAGNOSIS-RELATED GROUPS (DRGs)
(Continued)

DRG	MDC	TYPE	DESCRIPTION
366	13	Med	Malignancy, female reproductive system w CC
367	13	Med	Malignancy, female reproductive system w/o CC
368	13	Med	Infections, female reproductive system
369	13	Med	Menstrual and other female reproductive system disorders
370	14	Surg	Cesarean section w CC
371	14	Surg	Cesarean section w/o CC
372	14	Med	Vaginal delivery w complicating diagnoses
373	14	Med	Vaginal delivery w/o complicating diagnoses
374	14	Surg	Vaginal delivery w sterilization and/or D and C
375	14	Surg	Vaginal delivery w OR proc except steril and/or D & C
376	14	Med	Postpartum and post abortion diagnoses w/o OR procedure
377	14	Surg	Postpartum and post abortion diagnoses w OR procedure
378	14	Med	Ectopic pregnancy
379	14	Med	Threatened abortion
380	14	Med	Abortion w/o D & C

DIAGNOSIS-RELATED GROUPS (DRGs)
(Continued)

DRG	MDC	TYPE	DESCRIPTION
381	14	Surg	Abortion w D & C, aspiration curettage or hysterotomy
382	14	Med	False labor
383	14	Med	Other antepartum diagnoses w medical complications
384	14	Med	Other antepartum diagnoses w/o medical complications
385	15	Med	Neonates, died or transferred to another acute care facility
386	15	Med	Extreme immaturity or respiratory distress syndrome neonate
387	15	Med	Prematurity w major problems
388	15	Med	Prematurity w/o major problems
389	15	Med	Full term neonate w major problems
390	15	Med	Neonate w other significant problems
391	15	Med	Normal newborn
392	16	Surg	Splenectomy age >17
393	16	Surg	Splenectomy age 0–17
394	16	Surg	Other OR procedures of the blood and blood forming organs
395	16	Med	Red blood cell disorders age >17

DIAGNOSIS-RELATED GROUPS (DRGs)
(Continued)

DRG	MDC	TYPE	DESCRIPTION
396	16	Med	Red blood cell disorders age 0–17
397	16	Med	Coagulation disorders
398	16	Med	Reticuloendothelial and immunity disorders w CC
399	16	Med	Reticuloendothelial and immunity disorders w/o CC
400	17	Surg	Lymphoma and leukemia w major OR procedure
401	17	Surg	Lymphoma and non-acute leukemia w other OR proc w CC
402	17	Surg	Lymphoma and non-acute leukemia w other OR proc w/o CC
403	17	Med	Lymphoma and non-acute leukemia w CC
404	17	Med	Lymphoma and non-acute leukemia w/o CC
405	17		Acute leukemia w/o major OR procedure age 0–17
406	17	Surg	Myeloprolif disord or poorly diff neopl w maj OR proc w CC
407	17	Surg	Myeloprolif disord or poorly diff neopl w maj OR proc w/o CC
408	17	Surg	Myeloprolif disord or poorly diff neopl w other OR proc

DIAGNOSIS-RELATED GROUPS (DRGs)
(Continued)

DRG	MDC	TYPE	DESCRIPTION
409	17	Med	Radiotherapy
410	17	Med	Chemotherapy w/o acute leukemia as secondary diagnosis
411	17	Med	History of malignancy w/o endoscopy
412	17	Med	History of malignancy w endoscopy
413	17	Med	Other myeloprolif dis or poorly diff neopl diag w CC
414	17	Med	Other myeloprolif dis or poorly diff neopl diag w/o CC
415	18	Surg	OR procedure for infectious and parasitic diseases
416	18	Med	Septicemia age >17
417	18	Med	Septicemia age 0–17
418	18	Med	Postoperative and post-traumatic infections
419	18	Med	Fever of unknown origin age >17 w CC
420	18	Med	Fever of unknown origin age >17 w/o CC
421	18	Med	Viral illness age >17
422	18	Med	Viral illness and fever of unknown origin age 0–17
423	18	Med	Other infectious and parasitic diseases diagnoses

DIAGNOSIS-RELATED GROUPS (DRGs)
(Continued)

DRG	MDC	TYPE	DESCRIPTION
424	19	Surg	OR procedure w principal diagnoses of mental illness
425	19	Med	Acute adjustment reaction and psychological dysfunction
426	19	Med	Depressive neuroses
427	19	Med	Neuroses except depressive
428	19	Med	Disorders of personality and impulse control
429	19	Med	Organic disturbances and mental retardation
430	19	Med	Psychoses
431	19	Med	Childhood mental disorders
432	19	Med	Other mental disorder diagnoses
433	20		Alcohol/drug abuse or dependence, left ama
434	20		No longer valid
435	20		No longer valid
436	20		No longer valid
437	20		No longer valid
438			No longer valid
439	21	Surg	Skin grafts for injuries
440	21	Surg	Wound débridements for injuries
441	21	Surg	Hand procedures for injuries

DIAGNOSIS-RELATED GROUPS (DRGs)
(Continued)

DRG	MDC	TYPE	DESCRIPTION
442	21	Surg	Other OR procedures for injuries w CC
443	21	Surg	Other OR procedures for injuries w/o CC
444	21	Med	Traumatic injury age >17 w CC
445	21	Med	Traumatic injury age >17 w/o CC
446	21	Med	Traumatic injury age 0–17
447	21	Med	Allergic reaction age >17
448	21	Med	Allergic reaction age 0–17
449	21	Med	Poisoning and toxic effects of drugs age >17 w CC
450	21	Med	Poisoning and toxic effects of drugs age >17 w/o CC
451	21	Med	Poisoning and toxic effects of drugs age 0–17
452	21	Med	Complications of treatment w CC
453	21	Med	Complications of treatment w/o CC
454	21	Med	Other injury, poisoning and toxic effect diag w CC
455	21	Med	Other injury, poisoning and toxic effect diag w/o CC
456			No longer valid
457			No longer valid
458			No longer valid

DIAGNOSIS-RELATED GROUPS (DRGs)
(Continued)

DRG	MDC	TYPE	DESCRIPTION
459			No longer valid
460			No longer valid
461	23	Surg	O.R. proc w diagnoses of other contact w health services
462	23	Med	Rehabilitation
463	23	Med	Signs and symptoms w CC
464	23	Med	Signs and symptoms w/o CC
465	23	Med	Aftercare w history of malignancy as secondary diagnosis
466	23	Med	Aftercare w/o history of malignancy as secondary diagnosis
467	23	Med	Other factors influencing health status
468			Extensive OR procedure unrelated to principal diagnosis
469			Principal diagnosis invalid as discharge diagnosis
470			Ungroupable
471	08	Surg	Bilateral or multiple major joint procs of lower extremity
472			No longer valid
473	17		Acute leukemia w/o major O.R. procedure age >17

DIAGNOSIS-RELATED GROUPS (DRGs)
(Continued)

DRG	MDC	TYPE	DESCRIPTION
474			No longer valid
475	04	Med	Respiratory system diagnosis with ventilator support
476		Surg	Prostatic OR procedure unrelated to principal diagnosis
477		Surg	Non-extensive OR procedure unrelated to principal diagnosis
478	05	Surg	Other vascular procedures w CC
479	05	Surg	Other vascular procedures w/o CC
480		Surg	Liver transplant
481		Surg	Bone marrow transplant
482		Surg	Tracheostomy for face, mouth and neck diagnoses
483		Surg	Tracheostomy except for face, mouth and neck diagnoses
484	24	Surg	Craniotomy for multiple significant trauma
485	24	Surg	Limb reattachment, hip and femur proc for multiple significant trauma
486	24	Surg	Other OR procedures for multiple significant trauma
487	24	Med	Other multiple significant trauma

DIAGNOSIS-RELATED GROUPS (DRGs)
(Continued)

DRG	MDC	TYPE	DESCRIPTION
488	25	Surg	HIV w extensive OR procedure
489	25	Med	HIV w major related condition
490	25	Med	HIV w or w/o other related condition
491	08	Surg	Major joint and limb reattachment procedures of upper extremity
492	17	Med	Chemotherapy w acute leukemia as secondary diagnosis
493	07	Surg	Laparoscopic cholecystectomy w/o CDE w CC
494	07	Surg	Laparoscopic cholecystectomy w/o CDE w/o CC
495		Surg	Lung transplant
496	08	Surg	Combined anterior/posterior spinal fusion
497	08	Surg	Spinal fusion w CC
498	08	Surg	Spinal fusion w/o CC
499	08	Surg	Back and neck procedures except spinal fusion w CC
500	08	Surg	Back and neck procedures except spinal fusion w/o CC
501	08	Surg	Knee procedures w pdx of infection w CC

DIAGNOSIS-RELATED GROUPS (DRGs)
(Continued)

DRG	MDC	TYPE	DESCRIPTION
502	08	Surg	Knee procedures w pdx of infection w/o CC
503	08	Surg	Knee procedures w/o pdx of infection
504	22	Surg	Extensive 3rd degree burns w skin graft
505	22		Extensive 3rd degree burns w/o skin graft
506	22		Full-thickness burn w skin graft or inhal inj w CC or sig trauma
507	22		Full-thickness burn w skin graft or inhal inj w/o CC or sig trauma
508	22		Full-thickness burn w/o skin graft or inhal inj w CC or sig trauma
509	22		Full-thickness burn w/o skin grft or inhal inj w/o CC or sig trauma
510	22		Non-extensive burns w CC or significant trauma
511	22		Non-extensive burns w/o CC or significant trauma
512	Pre	Surg	Simultaneous pancreas/ kidney transplant
513	Pre	Surg	Pancreas transplant
514	05	Surg	Cardiac defibrillator implant w cardiac cath
515	05	Surg	Cardiac defibrillator implant w/o cardiac cath

DIAGNOSIS-RELATED GROUPS (DRGs)
(Continued)

DRG	MDC	TYPE	DESCRIPTION
516	05	Surg	Percutaneous cardiovascular proc w AMI
517	05	Surg	Perc cardio proc w non-drug eluting stent w/o AMI
518	05	Surg	Perc cardio proc w/o coronary artery stent or AMI
519	08	Surg	Cervical spinal fusion w CC
520	08	Surg	Cervical spinal fusion w/o CC
521	20	Med	Alcohol/drug abuse or dependence w CC
522	20	Med	Alcohol/drug abuse or dependence w rehabilitation therapy w/o CC
523	20	Med	Alcohol/drug abuse or dependence w/o rehabilitation therapy w/o CC
524	01	Med	Transient ischemia
525	05	Surg	Heart assist system implant
526	05	Surg	Percutaneous cardiovascular proc w drug-eluting stent w AMI
527	05	Surg	Percutaneous cardiovascular proc w drug-eluting stent w/o AMI

Normal Hematologic Reference Values and Implications of Abnormal Results*

The implications of abnormal results are major ones in each category. SI units are those used in the International System of Units, which generally are accepted for all scientific and technical uses. All laboratory values should be interpreted with caution because normal values differ widely among clinical laboratories.

cu mm = cubic millimeter (mm^3)
dL = deciliter (1/10 of a liter *or* 100 mL)
g = gram
L = liter
mg = milligram (1/1000 of a gram)
mL = milliliter
mEq = milliequivalent
mill = million
mm = millimeter (1/1000 of a meter)
mmol = millimole
thou = thousand
U = unit
µL = microliter
µmol = micromole (one millionth of a mole)

---

*From Chabner DE: The Language of Medicine, 9th ed. Philadelphia, Saunders, 2011.

BLOOD CELL COUNTS*

CELL CATEGORY	CONVENTIONAL UNITS	SI UNITS	IMPLICATIONS OF ABNORMALITY	
Erythrocytes (RBCs)				
Females	4.0–5.5 million/mm^3 *or* μL	4.0–5.5×10^{12}/L	*High*	• Polycythemia • Dehydration
Males	4.5–6.0 million/mm^3 *or* μL	4.5–6.0×10^{12}/L	*Low*	• Iron deficiency anemia • Blood loss
Leukocytes (WBCs)				
Total	5000–$10,000$/mm^3 *or* μL	5.0–10.0×10^{9}/L	*High*	• Bacterial infection • Leukemia • Eosinophils high in allergy

*From Chabner DE: The Language of Medicine, 9th ed. Philadelphia, Saunders, 2011.
RBCs, red blood cells; WBCs, white blood cells.

BLOOD CELL COUNTS (Continued)

CELL CATEGORY	CONVENTIONAL UNITS	SI UNITS	IMPLICATIONS OF ABNORMALITY	
Differential	(%)			
Neutrophils	54–62		*Low*	• Viral infection
Lymphocytes	20–40			• Aplastic anemia
Monocytes	3–7			• Chemotherapy
Eosinophils	1–3			
Basophils	0–1			
Platelets	150,000–350,000/mm^3 *or* μL	200–400 × 10^9/L	*High*	• Hemorrhage
				• Infections
				• Malignancy
				• Splenectomy
			Low	• Aplastic anemia
				• Chemotherapy
				• Hypersplenism

COAGULATION TESTS*

TEST	CONVENTIONAL UNITS	SI UNITS	IMPLICATIONS OF ABNORMALITY
Bleeding time (template method)	2.75–8.0 min	2.7–8.0 min	*Prolonged* • Aspirin ingestion • Low platelet count
Coagulation time	5–15 min	5–15 min	*Prolonged* • Heparin therapy
Prothrombin time (PT)†	11–12.5 sec	11–12.5 sec	*Prolonged* • Vitamin K deficiency • Hepatic disease • Oral anticoagulant therapy (warfarin)
Partial thromboplastin time (PTT)	25–34 sec	25–37 sec	*Prolonged* • Intravenous heparin therapy

*From Chabner DE: The Language of Medicine, 9th ed. Philadelphia, Saunders, 2011.
†The INR (international normalized ratio) is a standard tool for monitoring the effects of an anticoagulant, warfarin; the normal INR value is <1.5.

RED BLOOD CELL TESTS*

TEST	CONVENTIONAL UNITS	SI UNITS	IMPLICATIONS OF ABNORMALITY	
Hematocrit (Hct)				
Females	37%–47%	0.37–0.47	*High*	• Polycythemia • Dehydration
Males	40%–54%	0.40–0.54	*Low*	• Loss of blood • Anemia
Hemoglobin (Hb, Hgb)				
Females	12.0–14.0 g/dL *or* 120–140 g/L	1.86–2.48 mmol/L	*High*	• Polycythemia • Dehydration
Males	14.0–16.0 g/dL	2.17–2.79 mmol/L	*Low*	• Anemia • Blood loss

*From Chabner DE: The Language of Medicine, 9th ed. Philadelphia, Saunders, 2011.

SERUM TESTS*

TEST	CONVENTIONAL UNITS	SI UNITS		IMPLICATIONS OF ABNORMALITY
Alanine aminotransferase (ALT)	5–30 U/L	5–30 U/L	*High*	• Hepatitis
Albumin	3.5–5.5 g/dL	35–55 g/L	*Low*	• Hepatic disease • Malnutrition • Nephritis and nephrosis
Alkaline phosphatase (ALP)	20–90 U/L	20–90 U/L	*High*	• Bone disease • Hepatitis or tumor infiltration of liver • Biliary obstruction
Aspartate aminotransferase (AST)	10–30 U/L	10–30 U/L	*High*	• Hepatitis • Cardiac and muscle injury

*From Chabner DE: The Language of Medicine, 9th ed. Philadelphia, Saunders, 2011.

SERUM TESTS (Continued)

TEST	CONVENTIONAL UNITS	SI UNITS		IMPLICATIONS OF ABNORMALITY
Bilirubin				
Total	0.3–1.0 mg/dL	5.1–17 µmol/L	*High*	• Hemolysis
Neonates	1–12 mg/dL	17–205 µmol/L		• Neonatal hepatic immaturity
				• Cirrhosis
				• Biliary tract obstruction
Blood urea nitrogen (BUN)	10–20 mg/dL	3.6–7.1 mmol/L	*High*	• Renal disease
				• Reduced renal blood flow
				• Urinary tract obstruction
			Low	• Hepatic damage
				• Malnutrition
Calcium	9.0–10.5 mg/dL	2.2–2.6 mmol/L	*High*	• Hyperparathyroidism
				• Multiple myeloma
				• Metastatic cancer
			Low	• Hypoparathyroidism
				• Total parathyroidectomy

SERUM TESTS (Continued)

TEST	CONVENTIONAL UNITS	SI UNITS		IMPLICATIONS OF ABNORMALITY
Cholesterol (desirable range)				
Total	<200 mg/dL	<5.2 mmol/L	*High*	• High-fat diet
LDL cholesterol	<130 mg/dL	<3.36 mmol/L		• Inherited
				• Hypercholesterolemia
HDL cholesterol	>60 mg/dL	>1.55 mmol/L	*Low*	• Starvation
Creatine kinase (CK)				
Females	30–135 U/L	30–135 U/L	*High*	• Myocardial infarction
Males	55–170 U/L	55–170 U/L		• Muscle disease
Creatinine	<1.5 mg/dL	<133 µmol/L	*High*	• Renal disease

SERUM TESTS (Continued)

TEST	CONVENTIONAL UNITS	SI UNITS	IMPLICATIONS OF ABNORMALITY	
Glucose (fasting)	75–115 mg/dL	4.2–6.4 mmol/L	*High*	• Diabetes mellitus
			Low	• Hyperinsulinism • Fasting • Hypothyroidism • Addison disease • Pituitary insufficiency
Lactate dehydrogenase (LDH)	100–190 U/L	100–190 U/L	*High*	• Tissue necrosis • Lymphomas • Muscle disease
Phosphate (PO_4^-)	3.0–4.5 mg/dL	1.0–1.5 mmol/L	*High*	• Renal failure • Bone metastases • Hypoparathyroidism
			Low	• Malnutrition • Malabsorption • Hyperparathyroidism

SERUM TESTS (Continued)

TEST	CONVENTIONAL UNITS	SI UNITS		IMPLICATIONS OF ABNORMALITY
Potassium (K^+)	3.5–5.0 mEq/L	3.5–5.0 mmol/L	*High*	• Burn injury • Renal failure • Diabetic ketoacidosis • Cushing syndrome • Loss of body fluids
			Low	
Sodium (Na^+)	136–145 mEq/L	136–145 mmol/L	*High*	• Inadequate water intake • Water loss in excess of sodium
			Low	• Adrenal insufficiency • Inadequate sodium intake • Excessive sodium loss

SERUM TESTS (Continued)

TEST	CONVENTIONAL UNITS	SI UNITS		IMPLICATIONS OF ABNORMALITY
Thyroxine (T₄)	5–12 µg/dL	64–154 nmol/L	*High*	• Graves disease (hyperthyroidism)
			Low	• Hypothyroidism
Uric acid				
Females	2.5–8.0 mg/dL	150–480 µmol/L	*High*	• Gout
Males	1.5–6.0 mg/dL	90–360 µmol/L		• Leukemia

Internet Resources*

Patient education is a serious responsibility for health care professionals. Many health care facilities develop their own patient teaching materials. There also are groups, associations, businesses, and agencies that develop patient education materials for dissemination to the public. There are many tools that can be used to improve an individual's knowledge about a particular health care problem or issue. These include, but are not limited to, pamphlets, movies, video tapes, audio tapes, newsletters, and computerized instruction products. Information also can be supplied to the health care professional to develop materials. The names and addresses identified in the following listing are potential sources of information that have provided information for the *Miller-Keane Encyclopedia and Dictionary of Medicine, Nursing, and Allied Health*. Local chapters of national organizations also may be found in the telephone directory or on line and may serve as valuable resources for patient education material. Encyclopedias and directories of health-related associations constitute an additional source of information or contacts.

Alcoholics Anonymous

Website: http://www.alcoholics-anonymous.org

Alcoholics Anonymous (AA) is a fellowship of alcoholics who support each other to achieve and maintain sobriety. It is an unaffiliated, self-supporting group that collects no dues or fees and receives no outside funds. Its primary purpose is to carry the AA message to alcoholics who still suffer.

---

*Modified from Miller-Keane Encyclopedia & Dictionary of Medicine, Nursing, & Allied Health, 7th ed., revised reprint. Philadelphia, Saunders, 2005.

Alzheimer's Disease Education & Referral Center (ADEAR)

PO Box 8250
Silver Spring, MD 20907-8250
Phone: 800-438-4380
Fax: 301-495-3334
Email: adear@alzheimers.org
Website: http://www.alzheimers.org

The Center provides information about Alzheimer's disease, its symptoms and diagnosis, and Alzheimer's disease research supported by the National Institute on Aging. It offers a newsletter to health care professionals and other free publications to the public. Information specialists are available to answer questions about Alzheimer's disease by e-mail.

Alzheimer Society of Canada

20 Eglinton Avenue W., Suite 1200
Toronto, ON M4R 1K8
Phone: 416-488-8772
Toll-free (from Canada only): 800-616-8816
Fax: 416-488-3778
Email: info@alzheimer.ca
Website: http://www.alzheimer.ca

The Society is a national voluntary organization whose goals are to provide information and support to those affected by Alzheimer's disease and their families, to increase public awareness of Alzheimer's disease, and to search for a cause and a cure.

American Association for Homecare

625 Slaters Lane, Suite 200
Alexandria, VA 22314-1171
Phone: 703-836-6263
Fax: 703-836-6730
Website: http://www.aahomecare.org

The American Association for Homecare (AAHomecare) is the unified voice that represents all of the elements of home care under one roof—from home medical equipment and respiratory therapy to home health services and from rehabilitation technology to infusion therapy. AAHomecare is dedicated to the advancement of the value and practice of high-quality health care services at home.

American Council of the Blind

1155 15th Street N.W., Suite 720
Washington, DC 20005
Phone: 202-467-5081
Toll-free: 800-424-8666
Fax: 202-467-5085
Website: http://www.acb.org

The American Council of the Blind is a national membership organization established to promote the independence, dignity, and well-being of blind and visually impaired people. Services include a monthly magazine, the Braille Forum, subscriptions to which are available free of charge to individuals in the United States in Braille, large print, cassettes, and floppy disks.

American Dietetic Association

216 West Jackson Boulevard
Chicago, IL 60606
Phone: 312-899-0040
Toll-free: 800-366-1655 (Consumer Hotline)
Website: http://www.eatright.org

The American Dietetic Association (ADA) promotes the optimal health, nutrition, and well-being of the public. The National Center for Nutrition and Dietetics maintains a consumer nutrition hotline that provides information and referrals to registered dietitians throughout the country.

Amyotrophic Lateral Sclerosis (ALS) Association

ALS Association National Office
27001 Agoura Road, Suite 150
Calabasas Hills, CA 91301-5104

Information and Referral Service: 800-782-4747

All other services: 818-880-9007

Website: http://www.alsa.org

The mission of the ALS Association is to discover the cause and cure for amyotrophic lateral sclerosis (Lou Gehrig disease) through dedicated research while providing patient support, information, and education for health care professionals and the general public, and advocacy for ALS research and health care concerns.

Association of Community Cancer Centers

1600 Nebel Street, Suite 201

Rockville, MD 20852

Phone: 301-984-9496

Fax: 301-770-1949

Website: http://www.accc-cancer.org

The mission of the Association is to promote the continuum of high-quality cancer care (research, prevention, screening, early detection, diagnosis, treatment, psychosocial services, rehabilitation, and hospice) for patients with cancer and the community.

Asthma and Allergy Foundation of America (AAFA)

1233 20th Street N.W., Suite 402

Washington, DC 20036

Phone: 202-466-7943

Fax: 202-466-8940

Website: http://www.aafa.org

AAFA has been in existence for over 40 years and is a registered not-for-profit patient education organization dedicated to finding a cure for and controlling asthma and allergic diseases.

Bulimia Anorexia Nervosa Association (BANA)

300 Cabana Road East

Windsor, ON N9G 1A3

Phone: 519-969-2112

Fax: 519-969-0227

Email: info@bana.ca

Website: http://www.bana.ca

The objectives of BANA are to eradicate eating disorders; to promote healthy eating and acceptance of diverse body shapes; and to provide clinical, preventive, and advocacy services for people affected by eating disorders.

Canada Safety Council

1020 Thomas Spratt Place

Ottawa, ON K1G 5L5

Phone: 613-739-1535

Fax: 613-739-1566

Email: csc@safety-council.org

Website: http://www.safety-council.org

The Canada Safety Council is Canada's national not-for-profit safety organization. Its mission is to be a leader in the effort to reduce preventable deaths, injuries, and economic loss in traffic, work, home, community, and leisure environments.

Canadian Cystic Fibrosis Foundation

2221 Yonge Street, Suite 601

Toronto, ON M4S 2B4

Phone: 416-485-9149

Toll-free (from Canada only): 800-378-2233

Fax: 416-485-0960

Website: http://www.cysticfibrosis.ca

The purpose and objectives of the Canadian Cystic Fibrosis Foundation are to aid those afflicted with cystic fibrosis; to conduct research in improved care and treatment and seek a cure or control for cystic fibrosis; to promote public awareness through the dissemination of information using all forms of communication; and to raise funds and allocate same for the foregoing purposes.

Canadian Hard of Hearing Association (CHHA)
2435 Holly Lane, Suite 205
Ottawa, ON K1V 7P2
Voice phone: 613-526-1584
TTY: 613-526-2692
Toll-free: 800-263-8068
Fax: 613-526-4718
Website: http://www.chha.ca

The Canadian Hard of Hearing Association is the "voice" of the hard of hearing in Canada. CHHA is the only Canadian national nonprofit consumer organization run by and for hard-of-hearing people. CHHA exists to help the hard of hearing achieve independent, productive, and fulfilling lives.

Canadian Mental Health Association
2160 Yonge Street, Third Floor
Toronto, ON M4S 2Z3
Phone: 416-484-7750
Fax: 416-484-4617
Website: http://www.cmha.ca

The Canadian Mental Health Association is a national volunteer association that exists to promote mental health. CMHA's mission is operationalized through education, advocacy, research, service provision, and facilitation.

Canadian National Institute for the Blind (CNIB)
1929 Bayview Avenue
Toronto, ON M4G 3E8
Phone: 416-486-2500
Email: cnib@icomm.ca
Website: http://www.icomm.ca/cnib

CNIB is the world's largest provider of services to people with visual impairments and a global leader in adaptive and assistive technologies.

Cancer Care, Inc.
275 7th Avenue
New York, NY 10001
Phone: 800-813-HOPE
Website: http://www.cancercare.org

Cancer Care offers information, referral, individual and group counseling, and patient education free of charge.

Centers for Disease Control and Prevention (CDC)
1600 Clifton Road, N.E.
Atlanta, GA 30333
Phone: 800-311-3435
Website: http://www.cdc.gov

The CDC provides information on diseases, health risks, prevention guidelines, and strategies. A wide variety of services can be accessed through the CDC.

Clinical Reference Systems, Ltd.
335 Interlocken Parkway
Broomfield, CO 80021
Phone: 800-237-8401
Fax: 303-460-6282
Website: http://www.patienteducation.com
Contact: Sales Department

Clinical Reference Systems, Ltd. (CRC) offers software designed to generate patient education handouts in Windows and web-based formats in a wide variety of areas. Editing of topics and customizing of hand-outs are features.

The Combined Health Information Database (CHID)
7830 Old Georgetown Road
Bethesda, MD 20814
Website: http://chid.nih.gov

CHID is a cooperative effort among several agencies of the federal government. These agencies have combined their information files into one database, which has been available to the public since 1985. Topics are updated four times per year.

Crohn's and Colitis Foundation of Canada (CCFC)

60 St. Clair Avenue East, Suite 600

Toronto, ON M4T 1N5

Phone: 416-920-5035

Toll-free (from Canada only): 800-387-1479

Fax: 416-929-0364

Website: http://www.ccfc.ca

The CCFC is a national not-for-profit volunteer foundation dedicated to finding the cure for Crohn's disease and ulcerative colitis. To realize this, the CCFC is committed to raising increasing funds for research. The CCFC also believes that it is important to make all persons with inflammatory bowel disease aware of the Foundation, and to educate these individuals, their families, health care professionals, and the general public.

Cystic Fibrosis Foundation

6931 Arlington Road

Bethesda, MD 20814

Phone: 301-951-4422

Toll-free: 800-344-4823

Fax: 301-951-6378

Email: info@cff.org

Website: http://www.cff.org

The Cystic Fibrosis Foundation was established in 1955 to raise money to fund research to find a cure for cystic fibrosis and to improve quality of life for the 30,000 children and adults with the disease.

Endometriosis Association

International Headquarters

8585 N. 76th Place

Milwaukee, WI 53223

Phone: 414-355-2200

Fax: 414-355-6065

Toll-free: 800-992-3636

Website: http://www.endometriosisassn.org

The Endometriosis Association is a self-help organization dedicated to offering support and information to women with endometriosis, educating the public and medical community about the disease, and promoting and conducting research related to endometriosis.

Epilepsy Foundation

4321 Garden City Drive

Landover, MD 20785

Phone: 301-459-3700

Toll-free: 800-EFA-1000

Website: http://www.epilepsyfoundation.org

The Epilepsy Foundation is the national organization that works for people affected by seizures through research, education, advocacy, and service.

International Federation on Ageing (IFA)

380 Rue Saint-Antoine Ouest, Bureau 3200

Montreal, PQ H2Y 3X7

Phone: 514-287-9679

Website: http://www.ifa-fiv.org

IFA serves as an advocate for the well-being of older persons around the world. IFA is committed to providing a worldwide forum on aging issues and concerns and to fostering the development of associations and agencies that serve or represent older persons.

La Leche League Canada

Box 29, 18C Industrial Drive

Chesterville, ON K0C 1H0

Phone: 613-448-1842

Fax: 613-448-1845

Website: http://www.lalecheleaguecanada.ca

La Leche League Canada promotes a better understanding of breastfeeding as an important element in the healthy development of the baby, and through education, information, encouragement, and mother-to-mother support helps mothers nationwide to breastfeed. The main objective of La Leche League Canada is to help mothers breastfeed their babies.

Learning Disabilities Association of America (LDA)

4156 Library Road

Pittsburgh, PA 15234

Phone: 412-341-1515

Fax: 412-344-0224

Email: info@ldaamerica.org

Website: http://www.ldanatl.org

The LDA is an information and referral organization. The Association provides any and all information regarding learning disabilities in both children and adults. There are 500 chapters across the country. Persons who make contact with the LDA receive a free packet of material from the Association, which then refers them to one of its chapters. Membership also is offered.

National Asian Pacific Center on Aging

1511 Third Avenue, Suite 914

Seattle, WA 98121

Phone: 206-624-1221

Fax: 206-624-1023

Website: http://www.napca.org

The National Asian Pacific Center on Aging (NAPCA) is the leading advocacy organization committed to the well-being of elderly Asians and Pacific Islanders in the United States. NAPCA develops and administers programs to enhance the dignity and quality of life of its constituents. NAPCA provides a fax-on-demand service called FAX-IT that provides more than 300 pamphlets, brochures, fact sheets, and so on, in 15 languages on topics related to health, wellness, and social services. FAX-IT can be reached by dialing 206-624-0185 from any fax machine (telephone handset).

National Association for Visually Handicapped
22 West 21st Street
New York, NY 10010
Phone: 212-255-2804
Fax: 212-727-2931
Website: http://www.navh.org

The Association's primary goal is to promote hope, dignity, and productivity for those with uncorrectable visual impairments by encouraging the full use of residual vision through large print, visual aids, emotional support, educational outreach, advocacy, and referral services.

National Autism Association
1330 W. Schatz Lane
Nixa, MO 65714
Phone: 877-622-2884
Website: http://www.nationalautismassociation.org

National Clearinghouse for Alcohol & Drug Information (NCADI)
11426 Rockville Pike, Suite 200
Rockville, MD 20852-3007
Phone: 800-729-6686
TDD: 800-487-4889
Fax: 301-468-6433
Website: http://www.health.org

An agency of the U.S. Center for Substance Abuse Prevention, NCADI collects and distributes information about alcohol, tobacco, and other drugs to all interested persons. This clearinghouse provides a wide variety of free printed materials, as well as video tapes and disk-based products for a small cost-recovery fee.

National Clearinghouse on Child Abuse and Neglect Information
PO Box 1182
Washington, DC 20013-1182
Phone: 800-394-3366

Fax: 703-385-3206

Website: http://www.calib.com/nccanch

This clearinghouse collects, catalogues, stores, organizes, and disseminates information on all aspects of child maltreatment.

National Committee for the Prevention of Elder Abuse

101 Vermont Avenue N.W., Suite 1001

Washington, DC 20002

Phone: 202-682-4140

Fax: 202-682-3984

Website: http://www.preventelderabuse.org

The National Committee for the Prevention of Elder Abuse was established to promote greater awareness and understanding of elder abuse and the development of services to protect older persons and disabled adults and reduce the likelihood of their being abused, neglected, or exploited.

National Council on Alcoholism and Drug Dependence, Inc.

21 Exchange Place, Suite 2902

New York, NY 10005

Phone: 212-269-7797

Website: http://www.ncadd.org

The National Council on Alcoholism and Drug Dependence (NCADD) provides education, information, help, and hope in the fight against the chronic and often fatal disease of alcoholism and other drug addictions. Founded in 1944, NCADD, with its nationwide network of affiliates, advocates a threefold approach of prevention, intervention, and treatment and is committed to ridding the disease of its stigma and its sufferers of their denial and shame.

National Health Council

1730 M Street N.W., Suite 500

Washington, DC 20036

Phone: 202-785-3910

Fax: 202-785-5923

Email: info@nationalhealthcouncil.org

Website: http://www.nationalhealthcouncil.org

The National Health Council is a private, nonprofit association of national organizations that was founded in 1920 as a clearinghouse and cooperative effort for voluntary health agencies (VHAs).

National Institute of Nutrition (NIN)

265 Carling Avenue, Suite 302

Ottawa, ON K1S 2E11

Phone: 613-235-3355

Website: http://www.nin.ca

Founded in 1983, NIN is a private, nonprofit national organization in Canada dedicated to bridging the gap between the science and practice of nutrition and serving as a credible source of information on nutrition. The NIN also conducts and supports nutrition research.

National Institutes of Health

9000 Rockville Pike

Bethesda, MD 20892

Phone: 301-496-4000

Website: http://www.nih.gov

National Wellness Institute, Inc.

1300 College Court

PO Box 827

Stevens Point, WI 54481-0827

Phone: 715-342-2969

Fax: 715-342-2979

Website: http://www.nationalwellness.org

The National Wellness Institute has served professionals interested in wellness and health promotion since 1977. It focuses on professional education programs; resources and information dissemination through its professional association, the National Wellness

Association; and the development and distribution of lifestyle inventories and health risk appraisals.

The Nemours Foundation
The Alfred I. duPont Institute
1600 Rockland Road
Wilmington, DE 19803
Website: http://www.kidshealth.org

The Foundation maintains a very informative website known as KidsHealth.

Osteoporosis Society of Canada
33 Laird Drive
Toronto, ON M5S 3A7
Phone: 416-696-2817
Toll-free (from Canada only): 800-463-6842
Website: http://www.osteoporosis.ca

The Society educates and empowers individuals and communities in the prevention and treatment of osteoporosis. As a resource for patients, health care professionals, the media, and the general public, it provides medically accurate information on the causes, prevention, and treatment of osteoporosis.

Recording for the Blind and Dyslexic (RFB&D)
20 Roszel Road
Princeton, NJ 08540
Phone: 609-452-0606
Toll-free: 800-221-4792
Website: http://www.rfbd.org

RFB&D maintains the world's largest collection of professional resources and textbooks on audio tape for all academic levels. It serves people who cannot read standard print because of a visual, perceptual, or other physical disability.

SHARE Pregnancy & Infant Loss Support, Inc.
National Office
St. Joseph Health Center

300 First Capitol Drive
St. Charles, MO 63301
Phone: 800-821-6819
Fax: 314-947-7486
Website: http://www.nationalshareoffice.com

SHARE offers support to families and caregivers whose lives have been touched by the tragic death of a baby through miscarriage or stillbirth or in the newborn period by providing information, education, and a network of support groups across the country.

SIECUS (Sexuality Information and Education Council of the United States)

Publication Department
130 West 42nd Street, Suite 350
New York, NY 10036-7802
Phone: 212-819-9770
Website: http://www.siecus.org

SIECUS affirms that sexuality is a natural and healthy part of living. SIECUS develops, collects, and disseminates information, promotes comprehensive education about sexuality, and advocates the right of individuals to make responsible sexual choices.

Students Against Destructive Decisions (SADD)

255 Main Street
PO Box 800
Marlborough, MA 01752
Phone: 877-SADD-INC
Fax: 508-481-5759
Website: http://www.saddonline.com

Founded as Students Against Driving Drunk, this organization provides young people with the tools to address the problems of underage drinking, impaired driving, drug use, and their consequences.

United Network for Organ Sharing (UNOS)

1100 Boulders Parkway, Suite 500

Richmond, VA 23225
Phone: 804-330-8500
Website: http://www.unos.org

UNOS, under contract with the U.S. Department of Health and Human Services, is a nonprofit organization that administers the National Organ Procurement and Transplantation Network (OPTN) and the U.S. Scientific Registry of Organ Transplant Recipients mandated by Congress. It operates and maintains the national list of patients waiting for solid organ transplants. In addition, it maintains a computer-assisted system for allocating organs to people on the waiting list. The primary goal of the UNOS organization is to increase the number of donated organs. Through a number of strategies, including public and professional education, UNOS endeavors to bridge the gap between the number of persons waiting for transplants and the number of organs donated.

Information about organ donation and transplantation is available from UNOS 24 hours a day, 365 days a year.

PART 3

Body Systems Illustrations*

*Illustrations modified from Chabner DE: The Language of Medicine, 9th ed. Philadelphia, Saunders, 2011; and from Miller-Keane: Encyclopedia & Dictionary of Medicine, Nursing, & Allied Health, 7th ed., revised reprint. Philadelphia, Saunders, 2005.

Index of Body Systems Illustrations

This is an index of all of the important labels in the illustrations of the body systems. You can use it to locate the relevant illustration for a particular anatomic term you may have in mind.

CARDIOVASCULAR SYSTEM
(AORTA AND MAJOR ARTERIES)

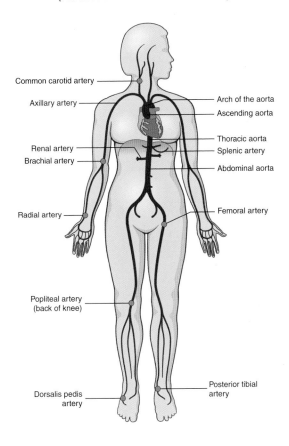

Common carotid artery

Axillary artery

Arch of the aorta

Ascending aorta

Thoracic aorta

Renal artery

Splenic artery

Brachial artery

Abdominal aorta

Radial artery

Femoral artery

Popliteal artery
(back of knee)

Dorsalis pedis
artery

Posterior tibial
artery

CARDIOVASCULAR SYSTEM (HEART)

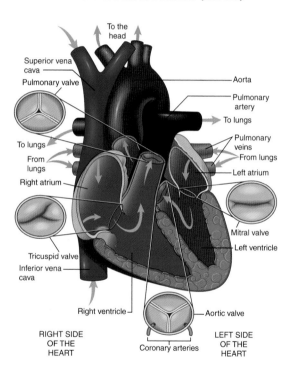

To the head

Superior vena cava

Pulmonary valve

Aorta

Pulmonary artery

To lungs

To lungs

From lungs

Pulmonary veins

From lungs

Left atrium

Right atrium

Mitral valve

Left ventricle

Tricuspid valve

Inferior vena cava

Right ventricle

Aortic valve

Coronary arteries

RIGHT SIDE OF THE HEART

LEFT SIDE OF THE HEART

DIGESTIVE SYSTEM

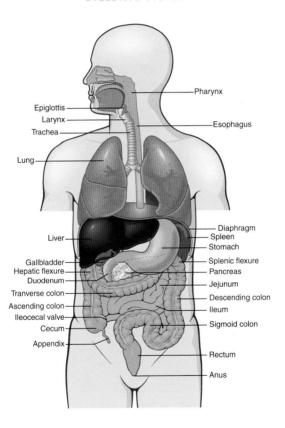

Pharynx

Epiglottis
Larynx
Trachea

Esophagus

Lung

Liver

Diaphragm
Spleen
Stomach

Gallbladder
Hepatic flexure
Duodenum
Tranverse colon
Ascending colon
Ileocecal valve
Cecum
Appendix

Splenic flexure
Pancreas
Jejunum
Descending colon
Ileum
Sigmoid colon

Rectum

Anus

325

EAR

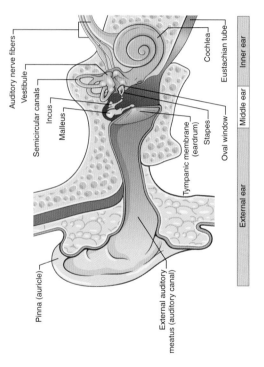

Auditory nerve fibers

Vestibule

Semicircular canals

Incus

Malleus

Cochlea

Eustachian tube

Tympanic membrane (eardrum)

Stapes

Oval window

Pinna (auricle)

External auditory meatus (auditory canal)

External ear | Middle ear | Inner ear

ENDOCRINE SYSTEM

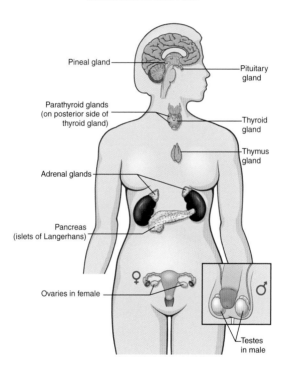

Pineal gland

Pituitary gland

Parathyroid glands (on posterior side of thyroid gland)

Thyroid gland

Thymus gland

Adrenal glands

Pancreas (islets of Langerhans)

Ovaries in female

Testes in male

EYE

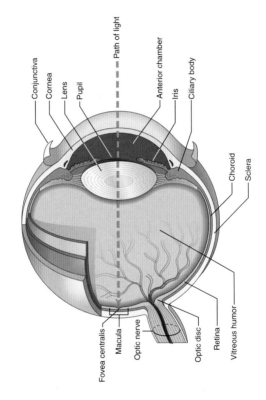

Conjunctiva
Cornea
Lens
Pupil
Path of light
Anterior chamber
Iris
Ciliary body
Choroid
Sclera
Fovea centralis
Macula
Optic nerve
Optic disc
Retina
Vitreous humor

INTEGUMENTARY SYSTEM (SKIN)

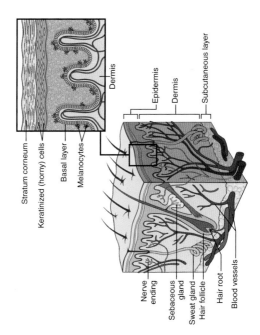

Stratum corneum

Keratinized (horny) cells

Basal layer

Melanocytes

Dermis

Epidermis

Dermis

Subcutaneous layer

Nerve ending

Sebaceous gland

Sweat gland

Hair follicle

Hair root

Blood vessels

LYMPHATIC SYSTEM

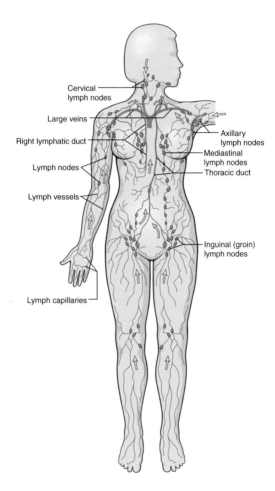

Cervical lymph nodes

Large veins

Right lymphatic duct

Lymph nodes

Lymph vessels

Lymph capillaries

Axillary lymph nodes

Mediastinal lymph nodes

Thoracic duct

Inguinal (groin) lymph nodes

MUSCLES (ANTERIOR SUPERFICIAL)

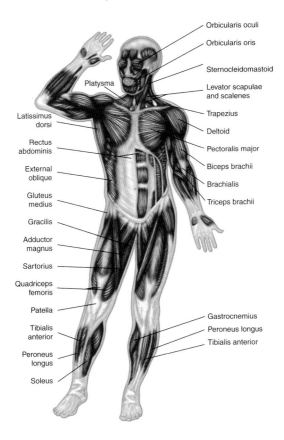

Orbicularis oculi

Orbicularis oris

Sternocleidomastoid

Levator scapulae and scalenes

Platysma

Trapezius

Latissimus dorsi

Deltoid

Rectus abdominis

Pectoralis major

External oblique

Biceps brachii

Gluteus medius

Brachialis

Gracilis

Triceps brachii

Adductor magnus

Sartorius

Quadriceps femoris

Patella

Gastrocnemius

Tibialis anterior

Peroneus longus

Peroneus longus

Tibialis anterior

Soleus

MUSCLES (POSTERIOR SUPERFICIAL)

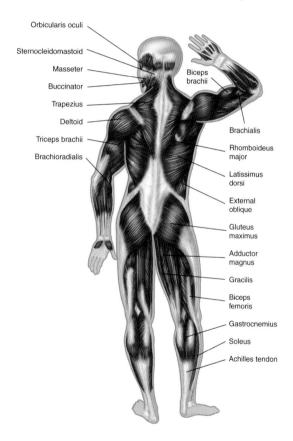

Orbicularis oculi

Sternocleidomastoid

Masseter

Buccinator

Trapezius

Deltoid

Triceps brachii

Brachioradialis

Biceps brachii

Brachialis

Rhomboideus major

Latissimus dorsi

External oblique

Gluteus maximus

Adductor magnus

Gracilis

Biceps femoris

Gastrocnemius

Soleus

Achilles tendon

NERVOUS SYSTEM

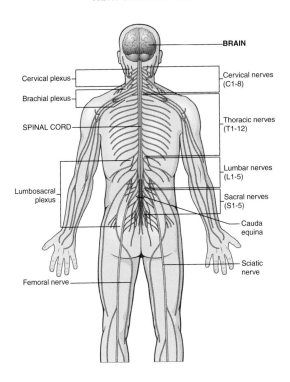

BRAIN

Cervical plexus

Brachial plexus

SPINAL CORD

Lumbosacral plexus

Femoral nerve

Cervical nerves (C1-8)

Thoracic nerves (T1-12)

Lumbar nerves (L1-5)

Sacral nerves (S1-5)

Cauda equina

Sciatic nerve

FEMALE REPRODUCTIVE SYSTEM

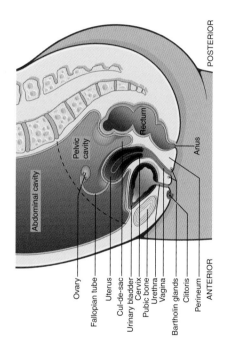

Ovary
Fallopian tube
Uterus
Cul-de-sac
Urinary bladder
Cervix
Pubic bone
Urethra
Vagina
Bartholin glands
Clitoris
Perineum

Abdominal cavity
Pelvic cavity
Rectum
Anus

POSTERIOR
ANTERIOR

MALE REPRODUCTIVE SYSTEM

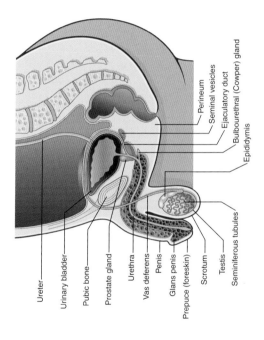

Ureter

Urinary bladder

Pubic bone

Prostate gland

Urethra

Vas deferens

Penis

Glans penis

Prepuce (foreskin)

Scrotum

Testis

Seminiferous tubules

Perineum

Seminal vesicles

Ejaculatory duct

Bulbourethral (Cowper) gland

Epididymis

RESPIRATORY SYSTEM

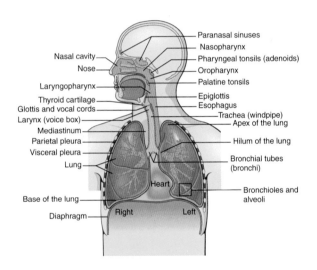

- Paranasal sinuses
- Nasopharynx
- Pharyngeal tonsils (adenoids)
- Oropharynx
- Palatine tonsils
- Epiglottis
- Esophagus
- Trachea (windpipe)
- Apex of the lung
- Hilum of the lung
- Bronchial tubes (bronchi)
- Bronchioles and alveoli

- Nasal cavity
- Nose
- Laryngopharynx
- Thyroid cartilage
- Glottis and vocal cords
- Larynx (voice box)
- Mediastinum
- Parietal pleura
- Visceral pleura
- Lung
- Base of the lung
- Diaphragm

Heart

Right   Left

SKELETAL SYSTEM

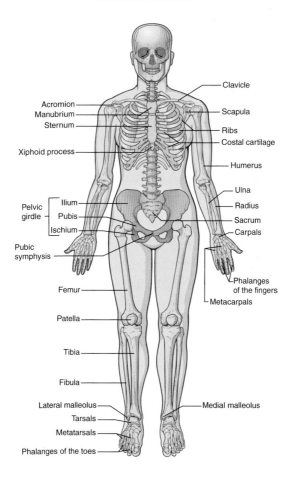

Clavicle

Acromion

Manubrium

Sternum

Scapula

Ribs

Costal cartilage

Xiphoid process

Humerus

Ulna

Radius

Pelvic girdle
- Ilium
- Pubis
- Ischium

Sacrum

Carpals

Pubic symphysis

Phalanges of the fingers

Metacarpals

Femur

Patella

Tibia

Fibula

Lateral malleolus

Medial malleolus

Tarsals

Metatarsals

Phalanges of the toes

URINARY SYSTEM

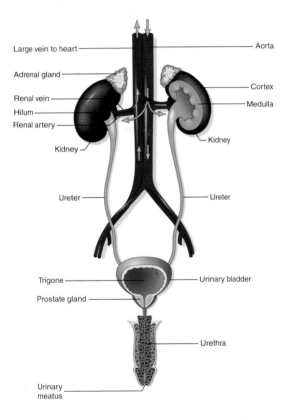

Large vein to heart

Adrenal gland

Renal vein

Hilum

Renal artery

Kidney

Ureter

Trigone

Prostate gland

Urinary meatus

Aorta

Cortex

Medulla

Kidney

Ureter

Urinary bladder

Urethra